Beat Obesity

YOU CAN IF YOU THINK YOU CAN

Teresa W. Blanc
Family Nurse Practitioner

ISBN: 1-4196-9480-4
ISBN-13: 9781419694806
Library of Congress Control Number: 2008902946

Visit www.booksurge.com to order additional copies.

"The first wealth is health."
— *Ralph Waldo Emerson*

Table of Contents

About the Author

Teresa W. Blanc, Family Nurse Practitioner, has compiled the knowledge and information about obesity and weight loss she has gained over the past fourteen years as a Nurse Practitioner into a concise, yet detailed book on weight management and goal setting.

Teresa received her Bachelor's Degree in Nursing from Missouri Western State University. She obtained her Master's Degree in Nursing with certification as a Family Nurse Practitioner from The University of Kansas and returned for a Post-Masters certification as an Acute Care Nurse Practitioner from Wichita State University.

As a Nurse Practitioner she has practiced in the Family Practice and Emergency Department settings, encountering many people with health issues related to obesity. Currently she is teaching at The School of Nursing at The University of Missouri-Kansas City.

Her vision: To help individuals achieve and maintain their optimal health status through education and training.

Her mission: To positively impact the lives and health of people everywhere.

You can reach Teresa at teresa@teresablancworld.com

Acknowledgement

I have encountered many people throughout my life that I have learned from, and it is these people I would like to take this time to thank for all they have taught me. First and foremost are my many nursing instructors. They have given me my knowledge and understanding of Nursing and taught me the value of good health.

Secondly, I would like to thank all the positive thinkers and motivational experts I have listened to and whose books I have read. Some of these are: Earl Nightingale, whom I listened to growing up as a young girl, Zig Ziggler, Brian Tracy, Roger Dawson, Andy Fuehl, Kerry Johnson and more. These are the people who have taught me the process of making and achieving goals and who I continue to listen to and learn from daily.

And two other very important people, who have provided the scientific theory needed to support the things I want to teach and share with people, are William Glasser, M.D., the creator of Choice Theory and Reality Therapy, and Robert Wubbolding, EdD, who has expanded on Reality Therapy.

To all these people I say, "Thank You." You have taught me so much.

A Word from the Author

Fifty million Americans will go on a diet this year. Many of these people will lose weight and keep it off for awhile only to regain the lost weight and perhaps even more. Many of these people have tried the weight loss systems and products on the market that have fabulous claims of effortless weight loss and are very disappointed with the results. Some develop diseases associated with weight loss products and medications.

Are you one of these people? If so, if you knew you could lose weight and keep it off, would you be willing to do what it takes to get there? If you knew that after applying what you learned you would see results and improve your health, would you try again?

That is what you are going to learn how to do when you read this book. You are going to learn mental, physical, and emotional strategies that others have successfully used to lose weight and keep it off and improve their health. You are going to learn how to take on the thoughts and habits of people who have achieved their weight loss goals. As you learn how to apply these principles to loosing weight you will also learn how to apply these principals to other areas of your life.

When you consistently use and apply the strategies, techniques, and skills you learn in this book, you will be able to transform your life, be healthier and happier, and enjoy doing things you long for or love to do for the rest of your life.

Are you ready? You can do it if you think you can. Let's get started now.

What have you got to lose?

Chapter One

The Pandemic

Obesity threatens to become the leading health problem of the 21st century. Obesity is referred to as a chronic disease and is the number one preventable cause of death in the United States next to smoking. It has been referred to as an epidemic and a pandemic. An epidemic refers to an outbreak of a disease of which there is a sudden, rapid spread. A pandemic refers to an outbreak of a disease occurring over a wide geographic area and affecting an exceptionally large portion of the population. Over 100 million Americans are overweight or obese. America is the fattest nation on earth with the other nations catching up quickly. Obesity is or is rapidly becoming a pandemic.

Many health risks and other diseases are associated with obesity. These include:

High Blood Pressure
High cholesterol
Insulin resistance and glucose intolerance
Diabetes
Heart Disease
Stroke
Gallbladder Disease

Gout
Osteoarthritis
Degenerative joint diseases
Obstructive Sleep Apnea
Respiratory diseases and disorders
Respiratory Failure
Complications of pregnancy
Poor female reproductive health
Bladder control problems
Kidney stones
Some types of cancers: endometrial, breast, prostate, and colon
Psychological disorders

More than four hundred thousand deaths per year are associated with obesity related illnesses.

As noted above, there are an estimated 100 million Americans overweight or obese. Statistics from 1999-2000 estimated that 64% of American adults are overweight or obese, as are 15% of children and adolescents. An estimated 50 million Americans will go on diets this year. Only 5% will manage to keep the weight off long term.

Obesity isn't just an American problem. Worldwide obesity has increased by more than 50% from 200 million to 300 million between 1995 and 2000.

In June, 1998 the first federal guidelines on obesity were released by the National Institute of Health. Overweight and obesity were defined by Body Mass Index (BMI). A

BMI between 25 and 29.9 is considered overweight. A BMI greater than 30 is considered obese.

What has caused this pandemic of obesity in the world? Obesity is a complex, multifactorial, chronic disease of malnutrition that develops from a combination of many factors including genetic, social, behavioral, cultural, physiological, and metabolic. No one thing alone can be said to cause obesity.

Originally the storage of fat in the body was a survival mechanism for humans. Fat was stored in the body for later use in times of famine. Rarely do we experience periods of famine in this country today. When we do it is usually related to a natural disaster such as a hurricane, flood, or tornado. Even when these things occur, the period of when people are without food is relatively short.

Today, instead of fat helping us to survive or live longer, some of us give up our lives early for it. Excess weight shortens our life span or decreases the number of years we have to live. Some of us give up our lives at an early age for hamburgers, cheeseburgers, and French fries. This can be compared to the person who gives up their life for cigarettes or the alcoholic who gives up his life for alcohol or the drug addict. In many respects, food is an addition just like the cigarettes, alcohol, or drugs.

A baby girl born today has a life expectancy of one hundred years old. However, if obesity continues to increase at the present rate, this may be the first generation to die younger than their parents.

In general, we have plenty of food today, and it is relatively inexpensive. In addition to our traditional foods we have processed food and fast food. All these types of food give us more choices as to what we eat, but all these types of food also mean we have excess food.

Environmental factors affect our weight. These factors include an abundance of energy dense foods, an increase in food consumption, larger portion sizes, fast foods and all you can eat buffets, inactive lifestyles, high fat diets, television shows, and advertisements promoting food. Smoking, marriage, stress, sleep deprivation and many more things related to our modern life styles affect our weight. Almost all our socialization activities today involve food activities of some kind.

It is interesting to look at how many of these environmental factors have changed over time. In America, food consumption has steadily increased, while physical activity has significantly decreased. We are now said to have a "sedentary lifestyle."

In 1970, Americans spent ¾ of their food dollar on food to prepare at home and about six billion dollars per year on fast food. This increased to around 110 billion on fast food by the year 2000. Today, a family spends about ½ their food dollars eating out at restaurants, many of which are fast food restaurants. An average American will consume approximately three hamburgers and four orders of French fries per week. Americans spend more today on fast food than they do for higher education.

In 1978 teenagers drank about one soda pop per day.

Today it averages three per day. Teenagers get as much as 10% of their daily caloric intake from soft drinks. A regular soft drink (not diet) contains about ten teaspoons of sugar. A teaspoon of sugar contains 15 calories. A twelve ounce soft drink contains about 180 calories from sugar. If a teenager drinks three, twelve ounce cans of soda pop per day this is 540 calories just from sugar! These are referred to as "empty calories" as they have no nutritional food value. Teenagers use to drink twice as much milk as soda pop. Now they drink twice as much soda pop as milk. Calories aren't the only problem. The extra calories cause weight gain, but excessive soda pop intake, especially in children, teenagers and women, can lead to calcium deficiencies and increased risk of bone fractures.

A generation ago, most food was produced on family farms and then sold to locally owned grocery stores. Meals were made "from scratch," meaning a recipe was used and food ingredients were put together to prepare a food dish. Today as much as ninety percent of our food is processed food, meaning it is raised and produced by big corporations where it is canned, frozen or dehydrated and mixed with flavorings and chemicals to make it taste good.

When food is processed, it looses much of it's nutritional value such as vitamins, minerals and fiber, and taste. Our taste buds and our sense of smell help us differentiate food that is good for us from food that is bad for us. Processed food has flavorings and chemicals added to make us think we are eating something good for us when it may not be. Processed food also has extra sugar and fat added, which makes more calories per serving. This makes our foods more energy dense. We also have many, many foods today that were not available a generation ago because of processing.

The food industry has developed a low-cost, dependable, very tasty food supply. Enough food is produced to provide each person in America with about 4,000 calories per day, and many of us eat that much. We only need about half that amount. If everyone consumed 4,000 calories per day, the average person would gain about twenty-four pounds per year. The average person doesn't gain that much, but there are people that do. A person weighing 500 or 600 pounds isn't that unusual anymore. There are whole industries being developed to provide clothing, furniture, medical devices, and other necessities for the obese person.

Food production has changed and increased due to technology as has our lifestyles. Food production has gone up and our activity levels have gone down. We sit in front of televisions and computers. We have all kinds of labor saving devices and more being developed each year. Foods that were considered a delicacy or a treat one hundred years ago are now everyday items. We have far too much food to eat for our activity levels, and our food has more calories per bite and taste better than at any other time in history.

Both husbands and wives work outside the home today. People are involved in many more daily activities outside the home than a generation ago. More meals are eaten out. Restaurant portions have gotten larger, and the food is richer due to competition and the marketing tactics used to lure people into eating at certain restaurants. Portions are "super sized."

Even food prepared at home has changed. More food is precooked and can be prepared by just heating it in the microwave. Many of our foods are "instant" as we just add water and heat.

We are taught to "clean our plates" when we are growing up. We learn we are suppose to eat all the food placed before us. Our subconscious doesn't let us forget this. We can still clean our plate. We just have to learn a few new guidelines on how to do it.

Food is everywhere today. Look around you. Almost every store has some type of food for sale. Gas stations used to sell only gas. Now they are convenience stores where we can grab something every time we go in. We don't use shopping lists anymore; we just pick food up as we need it. Little thought goes into the food value or how many calories the food has. It just has to taste good.

Building supply stores sell food. Office supply stores sell food. Vending machines are everywhere with soft drinks, candy, and snacks. Lunch rooms at schools are full of vending machines with this stuff (although some communities are putting a stop to these machines in schools). Even hospitals have franchised fast food restaurants instead of or in addition to a regular cafeteria.

I've heard people say that "at least you are in the right place when you have your heart attack." A popular song describes the "ninety-nine cent heart attack."

Food is advertised everywhere. You can't walk down the street, open a magazine, look on the internet, watch television, listen to the radio, or do many other things without seeing or hearing advertisements for food. Food companies have become the second largest advertisers in America. Automobile manufacturers are number one. We are told to eat twenty-four hours per day.

Not only is food available everywhere and all the time, but food is relatively cheap. This of course is due to technology. Food that is highest in calories and fat is often the cheapest food to buy. In the past, people in lower socioeconomic groups tended to have the highest percentage of obesity. This is changing. Obesity is a problem of all income groups today. It is also a problem of all age groups. Today there are two and three year old children weighing one hundred or more pounds.

Discrimination is a problem faced by the overweight and obese. Overweight and obese people are often discriminated against by insurance companies, employers, and by other people in general. Obese people may have trouble getting and keeping insurance and may be charged higher premiums. Insurance companies frequently will not pay for bariatric surgery that would help people lose weight although this seems to be changing as insurance companies are realizing the high cost of providing health care when the obese person does develop health problems or is hospitalized. Employers may not hire a person based solely on their weight and appearance; although they would never admit to this because of the possibility of a discrimination law suit. People in general may avoid the overweight or obese person. And these people are often the subject of cruel jokes and remarks by others.

If you are an overweight or obese individual, the focus of this book is to help you assess your current weight and health status and then to teach you about the power of choice and how to lose the weight you need to. You are going to learn how to evaluate your present weight , health status, behavior and actions related to controlling your weight. You are going to learn how to make goals and develop strategies and techniques to reach and maintain your goals. You are going to learn skills you can use the rest of your life to get to and maintain your weight loss goals, and the health status that you want and desire. The things you learn in this book you will be able to use for a lifetime, and you will be able to apply these skills to many other areas of your life.

First, you are going to learn about the digestive process and metabolism. Knowledge is power, and knowing how your body works gives you more power through this understanding. You are going to learn about many hormones that affect your weight and why. Then you are going to learn to develop a plan and the skills necessary to lose the weight you desire and to maintain this weight. So let's get started.

BEAT OBESITY

Destiny is not a matter of chance-
It is a matter of choice.
It isn't given to you, you earn it.

Only you control your destiny.

Chapter Two

Digestion, Metabolism, and Weight

After working in health care for many years now, I've discovered that people are much more successful in changing their health behavior if they understand what the body is doing and why it is doing it. I'm going to start with a brief summary of the digestion of food and how metabolism works in the body. I'm also including information about some hormones and other digestive substances in the body and their role in weight maintenance. I'm doing this to help you understand that weight loss is actually very complex. That is why there isn't one miracle food or drug that will solve all your weight loss problems. The information isn't going to be very exciting; in fact, some of you may consider it down right boring, but knowledge is power. Understanding what your body is doing and why gives you more power when it comes to developing your plan for weight loss and making your plan successful.

Digestion begins in the mouth. When you take a bite of food and chew it, the digestive process begins. Saliva in your mouth moistens the food to help break it down. The mucus membrane of the oral cavity actually begins to absorb sugar. That is why when a diabetic has a hypoglycemic reaction just putting some sugar in their mouth under their tongue will often bring them back to consciousness and increase their blood sugar level.

I've heard of some people "chewing and spitting" in an attempt to lose weight. Even when the food is spit out, some calories have already been absorbed. This is not a very satisfying way to loose weight. You will never get a feeling of satiety (feeling like you have had enough to eat) this way, and all of the good vitamins and minerals are being spit out while you are still absorbing the sugar and calories that you are trying to avoid.

After the food is chewed, it travels down the esophagus into the stomach. In the stomach, the food is mixed with gastric acid and hormones, which continue the digestive process and is formed into a mixture called chyme. The chyme then passes into the small intestine, where most of the nutrients are absorbed, then on into the large intestine. The large intestine completes the digestive process and the waste products are then passed out of the body through the rectum when you have a bowel movement.

This seems like a simple process, but while the food is passing through this long passageway, there are many other metabolic and hormonal processes occurring in the body that affects what is done with the calories, fiber, vitamins, and minerals that you have just consumed. Let's look at some of them.

First, what is metabolism? Metabolism is the process your body uses to determine how much you weigh, how much energy you need and have and how your energy is used. What kind of metabolism your body has determines the number of calories you need per day for your body to function properly.

There are a certain number of calories you need every day for your basic body functions like your heart beating, your breathing, and your movements. These are calories you burn just by being alive. This basic number of calories is called your *Basal Metabolic Rate* (BMR). You can compare your body to a car's engine; some run efficiently on a small amount of fuel, and others take lots of fuel to keep them moving. Everyone is different, but everyone has a BMR and a certain number of calories they must have daily. I'll show you how to estimate your BMR later.

Factors that affect your BMR are your age, whether you are male or female, your activity level, your genes (not jeans!) and your body shape. When you are young, you usually have a fairly high BMR. With a high BMR you burn calories easily. Males generally have a higher BMR than females. However, whether you are male or female, if you take in more calories than you burn, you will gain weight. As you get older, your BMR tends to decrease. If you don't adjust your eating habits, you will gain weight.

Calorie needs peak at about age 25 and then begin to decline by about 2 percent every ten years. One of the reasons for the reduced need is that as you get older muscle tissue in your body is replaced with fat, which (unfortunately) burns fewer calories than muscle tissue does.

There is an exception to the above information on calories needed. The exception is for women during pregnancy and breast-feeding. During these times calories should not be cut. A pregnant woman needs an extra 300 calories a day while pregnant and an extra 500 calories a day when breast-feeding. Consuming too few calories compromises a mother's health and the health of the baby.

Your body shape and size affect the number of calories you need. Muscle burns more calories than body fat does. So if you have a greater proportion of muscle to fat, your metabolism is higher. Likewise, if you have more body fat and less muscle, your metabolism is lower and you have a greater tendency to store fat than does someone who is tall and thin or someone who exercises regularly and has more muscle because of this.

A large person burns more calories doing an activity than a smaller person of the same sex and age. The more you weigh, the more calories your body uses. That's one reason men, who are usually bigger and weigh more than women, need more calories.

You have a genetic blueprint. The metabolic rate that you inherit from your family helps determine how many calories your body needs to function. Being a genetic factor, there is nothing you can do to change this. This is why your friend, who is the same height, weight, and activity level as you are, may be able to eat more calories than you and never gain weight. This is also one of the reasons you may have to work harder than someone else to lose weight.

Your activity level helps determine how many calories you burn. If you are active and burn more calories than you eat, you lose weight. If you are sedentary, get little exercise, and consume more calories than you use, you gain weight. The kind of exercise you choose, and how long and how intense you exercise, determines how many calories you burn. Some types of activity even help your body burn calories after you stop exercising. More about this later.

So how do you know what your BMR is? One quick and easy way to approximate your BMR is to multiply your current weight by ten if you are a woman, or by eleven if you are a man. Your body needs about ten to eleven calories for every pound you weigh to meet its basic needs. Additional calories are needed for all activity above those needed for the body to exist. This will be discussed in more detail when we get to the planning stage.

So now you have a basic understanding of the process of digestion and how your metabolism works. In addition to these, there are many, many hormones that affect your metabolism, your weight, and your appetite. The first hormones I want to discuss are the ones directly related to digestion, and then I will discuss the ones related to appetite and weight.

Your body has many glands that produce hormones and other substances. Hormones are chemical messengers that take their messages to specific parts of the body. There are two kinds of glands: exocrine glands and endocrine glands. Exocrine glands secrete their substances into a duct, which carries them to some body surface. For example, sweat glands carry sweat to the surface of the skin, where it is secreted through pores. Endocrine glands are glands of "internal" secretions of hormones. The gland secretes the hormone into the bloodstream. The hormone is then carried through the bloodstream to the appropriate area of the body where it is to do its job. The place the hormone is taken to is called a target organ, and a hormone is made so that it can only affect certain target cells. An example of this type of hormone is insulin, which is discussed below.

Many of these endocrine glands and much of our nervous system operate by negative feedback mechanisms. This means that high blood levels of a hormone or other substance will inhibit or stop further secretion of that hormone or substance.

Hydrochloric acid is one of the substances of digestion. When food enters the stomach, hydrochloric acid is secreted by the walls of the stomach. This acid helps break down food for digestion. This substance does not affect your appetite or weight except maybe indirectly if you develop a gastric ulcer or have problems with indigestion. Hydrochloric acid is the acid that makes your stomach and esophagus hurt if you have an ulcer or indigestion problem. Fortunately, the stomach is lined with a mucus membrane to protect itself from this acid. When the acid wears a hole through the mucus membrane, you can develop an ulcer.

As food passes into the first part of the small intestine, the duodenum, a hormone called Secretin is secreted into the bloodstream by the glands cells in the duodenum. Secretin was the very first hormone to be discovered. This hormone is carried in the bloodstream to the liver, the pancreas, and the stomach. The purpose of Secretin is to slow down the secretion of hydrochloric acid. So when hydrochloric acid travels from the stomach into the duodenum, Secretin tells the stomach to slow down the secretion of the hydrochloric acid. The hydrochloric acid is no longer needed after food leaves the stomach. It has done its job. The duodenum is not protected by the mucus lining that the stomach is. So when the Secretin arrives in the liver and Pancreas, sodium bicarbonate is released from the Pancreas to neutralize the hydrochloric acid in the duodenum. This prevents tissue breakdown in the duodenum.

Bile is another important substance that aids in the digestive process. Bile is a brownish-green, detergent-like substance made and secreted by the liver. It is carried to the Gallbladder where it is stored until it is needed. When needed, bile is carried to the duodenum, part of the small intestine, where it helps with the digestion of fats.

When you eat a large meal, especially one containing fat, the food bolus that passes from the stomach into the intestine and stretches the walls of the duodenum. A group of endocrine cells located in the duodenum wall are stimulated when the duodenum stretches and release a hormone called cholecystokinin (CCK).

CCK is a substance that stimulates the gallbladder to move. After the CCK is released, it is carried in the bloodstream to the gallbladder, where it stimulates the gallbladder to contract and release bile. The bile is then released into the duodenum, and the fat in the food is broken down into tiny fat globules. Once the fat is broken down into fat globules, the duodenum walls return to normal size, which stops the signal to release bile.

CCK also stimulates the pancreas to increase its secretion of digestive enzymes, amylase and lipase, into the duodenum. Amylase and lipase are enzymes which aid in the digestive process. Amylase is secreted into the duodenum to help digest starches and convert them to glucose to be used by the body. Lipase aids with the digestion of fat. Proteases are also secreted from the pancreas to help break proteins down into amino acids.

Insulin is another hormone produced in the pancreas in the section known as the Islets of Langerhans. Insulin helps you use the glucose from the food you eat. Much of this glucose is in the form of simple sugars. When you eat lots of sugar, the pancreas produces lots of insulin. The insulin is secreted into the bloodstream. The insulin helps the glucose cross cell membranes to be used by the cells. When you eat too much sugar, the pancreas has to work overtime to produce the extra insulin needed to metabolize the glucose. After a period of time, the pancreas can begin to wear out and become less efficient at producing the insulin you need, and you can develop type 2 diabetes mellitus. Type 2 diabetics do not produce enough insulin and eventually may not produce any insulin at all. Without the insulin the glucose cannot get into the cells, and a person will have a "high blood sugar" as well as other signs and symptoms of diabetes. These high insulin levels are referred to as hyperinsulinemia. Excess weight and obesity enhances many of the changes associated with hyperinsulinemia.

High insulin levels also promote changes in your blood vessels, especially the arteries. Insulin helps increase the formation of arterial smooth muscle cells. These smooth muscle cells make it easy for the accumulation of cholesterol plaque on the blood vessel walls, leading to peripheral vascular disease and heart disease, which increases our risk of heart attacks and strokes.

When you have high levels of insulin in the bloodstream, the liver senses this. The liver then secretes other enzymes (HMGCoA). Your body then starts to make substances that are part of the cholesterol family. These liver enzymes accelerate the conversion of calories into triglycerides and very low density lipoproteins (VLDL), which are two members of the cholesterol family. This is why many diabetics also have high cholesterol levels.

Not only are there changes in the pancreas as it attempts to produce more and more insulin, but tissues in the body, such as fat and muscle cells, become resistant to using the insulin properly and a condition called insulin resistance develops. When this happens, normal amounts of insulin are inadequate to produce normal insulin responses from fat, muscle, and liver cells. Glucose uptake is then reduced in the muscle cells, and glucose storage in the liver is reduced. Both these contribute to elevation of blood glucose. This effect also contributes to the development of type 2 diabetes and a condition called metabolic syndrome.

A syndrome is not a disease but a group of signs and symptoms resulting from a common cause or appearing, in combination, to present a clinical picture of a disease . Metabolic syndrome is characterized by a group of metabolic risk factors in a person. A person is considered to have metabolic syndrome if he or she has three of the following:

    a. Insulin resistance or glucose intolerance
    b. Abdominal obesity
    c. Hyperlipidemia
    d. Hypertension
    e. Elevated C-reactive protein
    f. High fibrinogen

If you consistently have a fasting blood glucose greater than one hundred, you may be insulin resistant. You are considered to have abdominal obesity if you are a woman with a waist measurement greater than thirty-five inches or forty inches if you are a man.

You are considered to have hyperlipidemia when you have a total cholesterol greater than 200, triglycerides greater than 150, HDL (good cholesterol) less than 60, and LDL (bad cholesterol) greater than 130.

Hypertension is a blood pressure greater than 140/90. The ideal blood pressure is less than 120/80, and you are considered to be prehypertensive if your blood pressure is between these two.

Elevated C-reactive protein is a proinflammatory state, and high fibrinogen is a prothrombotic state, both of which are determined through blood tests. If you think you may have metabolic syndrome, you should see your primary care provider to discuss this.

Another group of hormones associated directly with metabolism are the thyroid hormones. Approximately 20 million Americans have a thyroid problem, either hyperthyroidism or hypothyroidism. Hypothyroidism is more common and the one associated with increased weight gain by contributing to a low or decreased BMR. Half of these thyroid diseases are undiagnosed, and 80% are women.

The thyroid gland is located in the neck, and the hormones produced include Thyroid Stimulating Hormone (TSH), T3, and T4. The thyroid hormones help keep the metabolism of the body at the right speed. When thyroid levels decrease, cells throughout the body decrease in activity. When the cells are less active, they need less energy. This excess energy is stored as fat, and weight increases. In addition to weight gain, other effects seen on the body are slower heart rate, constipation, fatigue, feelings of being cold, dry skin, brittle hair and nails, hair loss, and decreased appetite even though weight increases.

People with normal thyroid glands have no problem burning excess calories to lose weight. People with underactive thyroid glands lose the ability to burn these extra calories. When a person with hypothyroidism consumes extra calories, these calories are stored, and weight is gained. The difference is the person with the underactive thyroid has a slower metabolism than normal, so fewer calories are needed for the body to function. The number of calories the person with hypothyroidism needs to survive may actually be very low. The person with a very low BMR may eat significantly less than a person with normal metabolism and still gain weight because he or she has lost the ability to burn these extra calories.

This is essentially the same thing that happens to a person who consumes an extremely low number of calories per day. The person thinks that the fewer calories he or she consumes, the more weight he or she will loose. This is true up to a point. There is a point where the body goes into "starvation mode." The body thinks there is not enough food available and it must conserve energy and use as few calories as possible. The body goes into a type of self-induced hypothyroidism and lowers it's own BMR for self-preservation, even though the thyroid gland may still be perfectly normal. These people will frequently be heard to say, "I hardly eat anything and I still gain weight," and their thyroid function tests are always normal. In this case these people must actually increase the amount of food they consume along with an increase in their activity level to raise their BMR so they can loose weight.

It is important that you get your thyroid levels checked before you start on a weight loss program. If you are having problems losing weight and your thyroid hormones are normal, then you know the cause of your not being able to loose weight is not a thyroid problem, and you will need to look for other causes for not being able to lose weight. You may need to talk with your health care provider about your concerns.

On occasion, I have had clients ask me to prescribe thyroid hormones for them to loose weight (to speed up their metabolism). Please DO NOT EVER do this. You might lose weight, but as soon as you quit taking the hormones you would probably regain your weight. But the real danger is in the potential development of osteoporosis (both women and men). Osteoporosis is a side effect of taking too much thyroid hormone, and a complication of hyperthyroidism. Osteoporosis is a bone disease that occurs as a result of loss of calcium from the bone. The bones become very thin and fragile. There is a very real increased risk of fractures, especially of the hip and lower extremities. It is very difficult to reverse this bone loss once it has occurred, sometimes impossible.

This has been a very brief discussion of a very complex system of digestion, metabolism, and weight. You may now be starting to realize how many of your bodily functions have to do with the intake of and metabolism of food. When you think about it, your body is very much like an automobile. The purpose of an automobile is transportation. The entire concept of the automobile revolves around the engine and the parts that work with the engine. In order for that engine to work and the automobile to function, you must provide the gas, the oil, the maintenance and upkeep for the automobile to perform efficiently. Your body has two main functions. One is intelligence so that you can think and make decisions for survival and to reach the goals you have in life. The other is providing transportation, so to speak, for you to perform the things your intelligence has determined you need or want to do. In order to provide you with this transportation, you have to provide the fuel and oil (food; nutrition) and proper maintenance for the body to function properly. Just as your automobile will last longer and you will get "more mileage" from it if you take proper care of it, your body will last longer and you will get "more mileage" (i.e. live longer and healthier) if you take care of it.

You've challenged your mind – now challenge your body.

Chapter Three

Gherlin the Gremlin and Other Hormones

The growing epidemic of obesity in the United States and the world has stimulated an interest in finding out what other factors might affect body weight in addition to the amount of sugar, fat, and calories consumed and the amount of exercise a person gets. As with digestion, what appears to be simple, the regulation of appetite, is actually another very complex issue.

Research has uncovered numerous hormones that play a role in appetite and weight. Some of these hormones help us loose weight, while others contribute to weight gain. Maybe one day, as a result of this research, there will be an effective weight loss medication or vaccination for weight control. I'm going to tell you about a few of these hormones and other substances... This should give you a whole new insight into the appetite you have and why it is sometimes so hard to control.

As you may have gathered from the previous chapter, hormones are very important to us. Hormones are the main regulators of metabolism, of growth and development, of reproduction, and of the stress response. Excess or deficits of hormones make the difference between normal and abnormal states in the body. Hormones can even make the difference between life and death in certain circumstances.

Your central feeding drive appears to originate in the hypothalamus, a structure in the brain. The hypothalamus is part of the nervous system. It releases hormones that affect digestion and appetite. It activates, controls, and integrates the peripheral autonomic nervous system, endocrine processes, and many bodily functions like temperature control and sleep.

Many of the hormones that affect metabolism and weight are called peptide hormones. These peptide hormones are just a class of hormones that work on specific cells called target cells. After the hormones are released into the blood stream, they begin the work they are designed to do once they reach their target cells.

The feeding drive is controlled by powerful satiety signals (the feeling of being full, having had enough to eat) that arise from orosensory stimulation (your mouth – food taste good), gastric distention (your stomach fills up and gets larger), and the interaction of nutrients with receptors in the small intestine as well as the hormones discussed below. Satiety occurs when you have the sense of being full.

You eat food because it taste good, and you are hungry. When you eat, food goes into the stomach, which expands, and eventually you feel full. When you feel full, you quit eating (maybe). When the stomach feels full, signals are sent to the brain to tell you to quit eating. When food leaves the stomach and passes into the small intestine, there are other signals sent to your brain to tell you to quit eating. This is one reason to eat slowly and chew your food well. Eating slowly allows time for the food to begin to pass into the small intestine and tell your brain you are full. This process takes fifteen or twenty minutes.

The infusion of nutrients from food into the small intestine is associated with the suppression of the desire for food. Interaction of nutrients with the small intestine stimulates the release of satiety hormones as well as slowing down the passage of food from the stomach. There is a purpose for this slow down. Most nutrients your body uses are absorbed in the small intestine. Therefore, this slow down gives you body time to absorb nutrients.

When you are hungry, your blood sugar is lower than normal and you have a hunger induced hypoglycemia. Carbohydrates provide energy absorbed in the small intestine. As this energy is absorbed your blood sugar rises, and the hunger induced hypoglycemia is reversed and you feel full. This hypoglycemia is normal and not associated with the hypoglycemia that affects people with diabetes when their blood sugar becomes too low. This hunger induced hypoglycemia is regulated within strict limits in the person without diabetes and periods of fasting normally will not be associated with the symptoms that affect diabetics. As your blood sugar rises, satiety areas in the hypothalamus are stimulated. This interaction between the intestinal glucose receptors, and hypothalamic stimulation may be one of the most important mediators of appetite as the result is decreased food intake.

A very interesting hormone produced in the stomach is known as ghrelin. I've labeled ghrelin as the gremlin. Ghrelin is produced by cells that line the stomach and when released, ghrelin stimulates appetitive. So those hunger pains you get may be ghrelin telling you to eat.

Ghrelin has been called the "first circulating hunger hormone." When ghrelin is released it stimulates the hypothalamus in the brain. The hypothalamus sends out signals that tell you, you are hungry and you need to eat. Put simply, gherlin increases food intake. Ghrelin levels increase before meals and during fasting. This makes sense as we are usually most hungry before meals and when fasting.

Have you or do you know anyone who works night shifts? Ghrelin levels have been shown to be higher from midnight to dawn and a lack of sleep stimulates ghrelin production. Perhaps this is why people who work night shifts report being hungry between midnight and five in the morning. It seems man times that night shift people weigh more than people who work day shift. Perhaps ghrelin has something to do with this. More about sleep later.

Interestingly, in research done with animals, ghrelin has been shown to potentially enhance learning and memory. The studies suggested that learning is best during the day and when the stomach is empty. Ghrelin levels are higher at these times.

After bariatric surgery, ghrelin levels decrease. This would make sense as a large portion of the stomach has been removed. This may help explain why people have very decreased appetites after bariatric surgeries.

When the body produces a hormone, there is usually another hormone that acts opposite of the original hormone to balance bodily functions. The hormone that balances ghrelin's actions is leptin. Leptin is a hormone produced in fat cells, circulates in the blood and enters the brain. Like ghrelin, leptin acts on the hypothalamus, but leptin works to reduce food intake. Therefore, leptin is a critical signal in the regulation of body fat and body weight.

Research is being done on both these hormones. There is still much to learn about these two. Some information available can't quite be explained yet. For example, weight loss results in decreased leptin levels, and obese persons have increased levels of leptin, suggesting obesity may be related to a decreased sensitivity to Leptin rather than a deficiency of Leptin. Leptin also seems to be affected by gender. Females secrete up to twice as much leptin as men.

Other hormones and genetic influences that affect weight include: cortisol, serotonin, dopamine, POMC, MC4R, obestatin, bobesine, neuropeptides, the Macagano gene and more. Briefly their effect on weight is as follows.

More is known about some of these than others, and research is ongoing in the hopes of finding a key to weight control that will help decrease the prevalence of obesity in the world today. I will discuss a few of these hormones.

One group of hormones is the melanocortin type hormones. These include adrenocorticotropic (ATCH) and melanocyte stimulating hormone (MSH) derived from prohormone-promelanocortin (POMC). Disruption of the melanocortin signaling system has been linked to obesity.

ATCH is a hormone produced by the anterior pituitary gland in the brain. It is released in response to low levels of circulating cortisol, stress, fever, hypoglycemia (low blood sugar), and major surgery. The signal for its release comes from the hypothalamus. It has a major effect on the metabolism of carbohydrates, fats, and proteins.

POMC is a substance needed for several of the peptide hormones to do their work. It is called a precursor hormone, meaning it necessary before the other hormones can be made. POMC helps activate the hormone Melanocortin-4 Receptor (MC4R) in the hypothalamus, which results in the suppression of food intake.

MC4R is a genetic peptide hormone from the pituitary gland essential for the maintenance of long-term energy balance. Its effect is through the hypothalamus.

When MC4R is activated in the body, you receive satiety signals from the brain, telling you that you are full. This hormone helps regulate signals in the hypothalamus with other areas of the central nervous system to regulate food intake and energy expenditure. When fat storage is increased, MC4R is stimulated and our appetite decreases. If fat storage is decreased (you are loosing weight), MC4R is not stimulated and your appetite increases.

A percentage of childhood obesity (2 to 6%) has been linked to a genetic mutation of the MC4R gene. Although this is very rare, if identified early and with aggressive treatment, childhood obesity may be prevented. Mutation of this gene is one of about six different genetic forms of childhood obesity. There is ongoing research on this type of obesity. Genetic testing is the only method for definite diagnosis of a MC4R deficiency.

Please note that childhood obesity, like all obesity, is a multifactorial disease that may be genetically and environmentally linked. A deficiency of MC4R can affect a child's ability to sense when they are full. Knowing this might help parents understand the child's eating behavior. The parents might then be able to develop techniques to decrease the child's intake of food and make other lifestyle modification to help control the child's weight.

Corticotropin releasing hormone is made by the paraventricular neurons in the brain. It contributes to the reduction of food intake and may be involved in stress and illness.

Cortisol is one of the steroid hormones in the body called glucocorticoids. Glucocorticoids are involved in the control of body weight. Cortisol helps us handle stress. When our stress levels go up, receptors in the hypothalamus are stimulated and cortisol levels go up. Some research studies have shown that excess cortisol contributes to the deposition of fat in the abdominal region as well as increased blood pressure, suppressed immune function and impaired wound healing. Excessive cortisol production can lead to signs and symptoms of Cushings Disease. It is known that people with more abdominal fat are at higher risk for cardiovascular disease.

There are many over-the-counter food supplements that claim to fight obesity by decreasing cortisol levels. Research has not proven this. Even if it did, with the multiple controls in our body that contribute to the regulation of weight, it would probably not be very effective. There is no simple answer for the treatment of obesity. Cortisol levels are not increased in obesity; they are increased when stress increased. The fact that someone is obese has nothing to do with his or her cortisol levels. And why would you want to decrease a hormone that helps us handle stress?

It is my recommendation that you don't self-medicate with hormones or other drugs where you could potentially do yourself more harm than good.

Decrease your cortisol levels by exercise and relaxation techniques that are proven to help reduce stress levels. Do this and not only will you have decreased stress levels, but you will burn extra calories which will help you loose weight.

Choleycystichinine is released in response to eating and plays an important role in meal termination. When combined in the system with glucogon, it helps produced feelings of satiety.

Bobesine is a gastrointestinal peptide that acts on the body and brain to produce satiety. It plays a part in the release of choleysystichinine.

Neuropeptide Y is the most widely distributed neuropeptide in the brain. It is one of the most potent appetite stimulators. It appears to have a role in the action of leptin in the brain. There is much interest and research going on concerning the identification of Neuropeptide Y subtypes and their effect on food intake and energy balance.

Two subtypes of Neuropeptide Y are Y1 and Y5. Research suggests that decreased Y1 and Y5 may cause obesity by blocking MC4R receptors, which decrease food intake thus doing the opposite and causing increased food intake.

Serotonin is a hormone that affects mood. It helps determine if you are in a good mood or bad mood, happy or depressed. Many of the newer antidepressants affect Serotonin levels. Research has been done in an attempt to use these drugs for weight loss. Some have initially helped people loose weight but then have worked the opposite and caused weight gain.

Carbohydrate consumption increases serotonin levels and helps make us feel good. This is why high carbohydrate foods are known as "comfort foods." Carbohydrates elevate your mood. Chocolate is known to be a "natural mood elevator."

Obestatin is a newly discovered peptide hormone. Research carried out at the Stanford University School of Medicine in 2005 identified this new hormone. It appears to be related to ghrelin. It is produced in the cells lining the stomach and small intestine. Research show it reduces appetite in mice. Research is ongoing to see if it has the same effect in humans, which it is believed it does.

DHEA (dehydroepiandrosterone) is a natural steroid hormone produced from cholesterol by the adrenal glands. You may have seen this drug promoted as a "miracle weight loss drug." Research shows that DHEA can be effective in controlling obesity in rats and mice but has never been shown to do the same for humans. Very little is known about the long term effects of this drug and what the side effects might be. Other studies show that DHEA may be of benefit in cardiovascular disease, some cancers, osteoporosis and others. I would not recommend this drug until more is known about its beneficial and harmful effects.

A recently identified gene associated with weight control is the Macagano gene. It is thought to be a obesity suppressor gene. So far only animal research has been done and results are preliminary.

Hormones and genes aren't the only things that affect weight. We've already noted some of the effects of our modern lifestyle on our weight. Our lifestyles also affect our sleep patterns and research shows our sleep patterns and the amount of sleep we get affects our weight.

One would think that if you are awake longer, you would burn more calories as our BMR goes down when we sleep. However, studies show that people who get less than four hours sleep per night are 73% more likely to be obese; those who get less than five hours sleep per night are 50% more likely, and those who get less than six hours are 23% more likely to be obese than people who get an average of eight or nine hours sleep per night. Sleep regulates hormones and other bodily processes. We need this eight or nine hours sleep for the body to function properly.

Getting less than the recommended eight or nine hours sleep has an effect on many of the hormones that control weight. Leptin levels go down, and grehlin levels go up with sleep deprivation. When leptin levels go down, appetite increases. Glucose metabolism and serotonin release are also affected by sleep deprivation. Decreased serotonin levels lead to carbohydrate cravings. Cortisol levels are affected as sleep deprivation causes increased stress on the body. Judgment and the ability to make good decisions are negatively affected when sleep time is shortened, which contributes to overeating.

Studies also show that people who are sleep deprived tend to get less physical activity, especially daytime physical activity. Less physical activity means you will burn fewer calories.

Lack of sleep is one area I can personally relate to. As a nurse, I have worked my share of night shifts. I know that when I worked at night I averaged two to three hours less sleep per 24 hours than when I work during the day. I also know that I snacked much more during a night shift than I ever did during a day shift and part of the snacking was to try to stay awake. At 4:00 or 5:00 a.m., I always had an intense urge to eat (and did). Also, when I worked night shifts I did not get my daily walking and other physical activity that I normally would have.

Obesity itself interferes with sleep. As weight goes up there is an increase in the risk of developing Obstructive Sleep Apnea (OSA). As weight increases the anatomy of the pharyngeal airway is altered by the adipose or fat tissue that accumulates in this area. This may not be apparent during the day when the individual is in an upright position, but when lying flat, the excess tissue occludes the airway, which interrupts the sleep cycle causing sleep deprivation.

Not only do hormones, genes, stress and sleep affect weight, but research shows that even our taste buds can affect our weight. You may never have thought about your taste buds affecting your weight. Taste buds are on your tongue. The tongue has about ten thousand taste buds with taste sensations for salt, sour, sweet, and bitter. Originally, it was thought that different parts of the tongue were specific for specific tastes. The theory now is that taste buds are in clusters of fifty to one hundred cells and can respond to all types of taste.

Tasting food is actually a combination of smell and taste. An assortment of things affect our taste buds and sense of smell. Examples are cigarette smoke, a common cold or sinus infection, allergies, and medications. All of these things can contribute to a loss of taste and smell and therefore a loss of appetite. Even our age affects our sense of taste. Both the sense of smell and the sense of taste decline as we get older. This leads to decreased appetite as we get older.

Taste buds are the body's natural mechanism for accepting or rejecting the foods we eat. Research shows that we are not only driven to eat by hunger but by the palatability of food. When we are hungry and have "cravings" for certain foods, our taste buds may be contributing to the desire for a certain food. Studies show that when we satisfy our cravings for a certain food by eating the food, the sensitivity of the taste buds is reduced significantly.

It has also been suggested that our taste buds change over a period of time. This might account for our likes and dislikes of food at different ages. For example, a five year girl old may absolutely refused to eat broccoli. The food may even make the child throw up. This same child may develop "a taste" for broccoli as an adult, and broccoli may become one of one of her favorite foods. So our taste buds could play a part in leading us to eat foods that make us obese as well as lead us to foods that help us stay healthy.

Perhaps we can play a part in changing what foods our taste buds make us crave. By eating foods that are good for us and lower in fat, higher in fiber, and by eating more fruits and vegetables we might be able to "train" our taste buds to want these foods that will help keep us healthy. Over time this could have a significant effect on our weight for the better.

Recent research by the Mount Sinai School of Medicine has identified taste receptors in the human intestines. The taste receptors discovered appear to be critical to sweet taste on the tongue and are involved with the sense of glucose in the intestine which would affect the secretion of insulin and other hormones that regulate appetite. It will be interesting to see what further research shows on this subject.

As you can see, there are many, many hormones, genes and other substances in the body that affect weight. Hopefully, you are beginning to realize why all the products that claim to be "miracle cures" for obesity will most likely be ineffective for permanent weight loss. Also, with all the research that is being done in regards to obesity, it is highly unlikely that any product that really works is going to be an over the counter drug when it is found. It will be a prescription drug, and there will most likely be strict guidelines for dispensing it. In the past, many weight loss drugs that were thought to be safe, both prescription and over-the -counter drugs, were found to be associated with deadly diseases such as Pulmonary Hypertension and were taken off the market. My pharmacology professor used to say, "Medicines are poisons with therapeutic side effects." The longer I prescribe medications, the more I realize how right he was, especially medications relating to weight loss.

All of this research and all the discoveries are important. Research is turning up more and more information that will eventually lead to some type of successful weight loss product. But even when that occurs, unless you know how to control your intake of food and your activity level, weight loss will not be permanent. So read on. The best is yet to come.

Plan + discipline = success

Luck = preparation + opportunity

Chapter Four

Proteins, Carbs and Cabbage Soup

There isn't a day that goes by that I don't have two or three emails urging me to try this or that new diet that is suppose to make me lose weight effortlessly, while I'm sleeping, or while I eat all the food I want. It seems as if every magazine on the market has advertisements for these diets or for food supplements that help you accomplish these things "without dieting" or by some special diet with special foods. These are just fads or gimmicks to sell products. Some of them do work, but when you return to your normal eating habits so does the weight. These things are sometimes referred to as "fad diets."

The definition of a fad is "a practice or interest followed for a time with exaggerated zeal." Isn't that exactly what happens with these diets? We read or hear about them for a period of time and then they seem to vanish. If they work so well, why don't they continue to be promoted and used?

This isn't to say that there aren't some good weight loss programs out there because there are, but frequently these diets advise you to eat a certain food or nutrient, or combination of foods for easy weight loss.

These diets work because they are low in calories not because of the magic of a certain food. Get your nutrition book and look up the calories for the foods that are suggested. Often these will add up to less than a thousand calories per day.

In addition to being low in calories many of these diets are not well-balanced. Many cause nutritional deficiencies. The famous "Cabbage Soup Diet" even warns people not to stay on the diet for more than a few weeks because of the risk of malnutrition.

Fad diets do not teach eating habits that are important for long-term weight management and good health. Avoid diets that focus only on certain foods or nutrients and don't consider the total diet. To lose weight and maintain weight loss you must choose an eating plan you can live with. You must make healthy food choices, learn how to prepare healthy food, and learn weight management strategies. Planning and careful food selection will ensure that your diet is nutritionally adequate and health risks are minimal. This type of diet can be continued long term without fear of nutritional deficiency and harmful effects on your body.

Your weight loss strategies must be accompanied by behavior changes and exercise training. Your diet must provide satiety to ensure you feel full after eating. Your diet must be one you can live with to maintain your goal weight.

The average American adult consumes approximately 2,300 calories per day, which is more than most need.

Weight loss is a function of creating an energy deficit, meaning a hypocaloric diet. Hypocaloric is a word meaning you are consuming fewer calories than you need to maintain your body weight. You will not lose weight unless you eat fewer calories than you use. Generally a deficit of five hundred to one thousand calories per day is needed to loose weight.

Some people diet by skipping meals. The "Skip a Meal Diet." In fact, more than 90% of dieters skip meals in an attempt to save on calories. One of the most frequently skipped meals is breakfast. People who skip breakfast have metabolic rates 4 to 5% below those who eat breakfast. Research shows that people who eat breakfast actually eat less and burn more calories throughout the day than those who skip breakfast. Don't skip meals, just eat smaller portions. Appetite expands or shrinks with your stomach. Eating less at one meal sitting will shrink your stomach and help you feel full sooner. If you get hungry before your next meal, eat a low calorie, low energy dense , healthy snack.

Other popular diets are very low calorie diets, low fat diets, low carb diets, high protein diets, formula diets and special foods diets. There are pros and cons to each of these.

A very low calorie diet is a diet less than eight hundred calories per day. These diets should not be used for more than two weeks and any diet resembling this needs to be managed by a health care provider. These should only be used by those with a BMI of greater than thirty or with comorbidities (having more than one chronic disease process affecting your body). These diets should NEVER be used by pregnant or breast feeding women, children or adolescents.

A very low calorie diet should only be a temporary diet used to induce large, rapid weight loss under medical supervision. The health care provider should evaluate each case individually to determine if a very low calorie diet is really needed for the person. Vitamin and mineral supplements must be included. People generally lose three to five pounds per week on these diets until their metabolism slows down. Then the weight slows tremendously or they quit losing altogether and can even gain weight due to the slow down in the metabolic rate.

People on very low calorie diets generally are not hungry after the first few days. This is due to the body being in a "ketogenic state." Another name for this type of diet is "therapeutic anorexia." This type of diet is often used to jump start a weight loss program. Regular food is slowly reintroduced into the diet. When the person returns to their previous eating habits, the weight may be regained quickly.

Side effects of very low calorie diets include fatigue, constipation, and nausea and vomiting. The most serious side effect is the formation of gallstones. This happens for a couple of reasons. First, you may already have gallstones and not know it. Rapid weight loss may cause these gallstones to produce symptoms. Second, rapid weight loss may cause a decrease in gallbladder contractions. If the gallbladder does not contract often enough to empty bile out of the gallbladder, gallstones may form.

Many people go on a "low fat diet." On a low fat diet you are limiting the amount of fat in your diet. Fat contains nine calories per gram compared to four calories per gram for carbohydrates. So decreasing the amount of fat in your diet does help you reduce the number of calories you consume. What frequently happens though is when people go on a low fat diet they end up replacing the high fat foods with too many carbohydrate containing foods. Your body needs carbohydrates to function properly but consuming too many will only replace the calories that were in the high fat foods. The high fat foods need to be replaced with complex carbohydrates, fruits, vegetables, and other high fiber foods. (See appendix for examples of each type of food).

Remember though that fat, like other vitamins and minerals, is an essential food component. You need a certain amount of fat in your diet to survive. Fats also help satisfy hunger and help you know when to stop eating. Often eating something with just a little fat in it will be enough to tell your body it is full and time to stop eating.

There are good fats and bad fats. Saturated fats are the bad fats and unsaturated fats are the good fats. Begin to look at food labels and learn which foods and food products contain saturated and unsaturated fats. Learn to choose foods with the unsaturated fats.

Many people are convinced that low carbohydrate diets are the way to go. Carbohydrates aren't the bad guys that they are made out to be. Like other food nutrients, they are essential part of a balanced diet.

Like fat, there are good carbs and bad carbs. Simple or refined carbohydrates are the bad carbs, and complex carbohydrates are the good carbs. A simple carbohydrate is one that is made up of one or two sugar molecules. A complex carbohydrate is one made up of chains of three or more single sugar molecules linked together.

Simple or refined carbohydrates are found in many processed foods that we eat today. Think of these as high sugar containing foods. Examples of these carbs are baked goods, breads, snack foods, convenience foods, candy, cookies, and other sweets. These refined, or simple, carbohydrates are the ones to limit your intake of. These carbs cause rapid changes in blood sugar levels, which stimulates hunger and encourages you to overeat.

Complex carbohydrates should make up about half of your daily caloric intake. Examples of complex carbohydrates are fruits, vegetables, beans, legumes, nuts, seeds, and high fiber foods. What makes the difference in these two groups of carbohydrates is the fiber.

Our modern food processing removes the fiber from these foods. Once the fiber is gone, the way these foods are digested and metabolized in the body changes, and this leads to weight gain. Once the fiber is gone, the foods are broken down into simple sugars. Fiber in food is not broken down into sugar. Because the fiber isn't broken down it slows carbohydrate digestion to help keep blood sugar levels low. Fiber also carries waste and toxins out of your body which helps to lower LDL cholesterol, prevent constipation, and aid in the prevention of colon cancer. More about fiber later.

Just as there are minimum daily requirements for vitamins and minerals, there are minimum daily requirements for carbs. The body requires a minimum of 100 grams of carbohydrate per day to ensure that fat is utilized properly, the brain functions properly, and that glucose is utilized properly. So the kind of carbohydrate that you eat is what is important. Carbohydrates are part of a balanced diet, and you need them to live healthily.

When people talk about carbohydrates, they often refer to the "Glycemic Index." This index measures the degree to which eating a certain food increases blood sugar and therefore contributes to weight gain. There are "Glycemic Index" charts just as there are calorie charts. These charts can be found on the web or in books.

When using the Glycemic Index as a guide in choosing foods, concentrate on eating foods with a low Glycemic Index. These foods will include more of your fruits and vegetables and whole grain product. Foods with a high Glycemic index stimulate short term appetite and lead to overeating. The higher the Glycemic index, the shorter term the satiety. Glycemic Index is not usually listed on nutritional labels. Become familiar with the Glycemic index of foods to help you make better food choices.

Complex carbs add satiety to a meal. This is a good thing as this satiety feeling helps slow digestion rates. When this happens, insulin levels rise moderately rather than rapidly and remain sustained for a longer period of time. This contributes to appetite suppression.

Carbohydrates are sometimes referred to as "comfort foods." They are associated with mood elevation. They make you feel good. High carbohydrate, low protein diets are the ones associated with this mood elevation. What happens is that the carbs stimulate the pancreas to secret insulin. When this happens amino acids in the blood are decreased. This increases the level of a substance called Tryptophane, which goes to the brain. When the Tryptophan goes to the brain, there is an increase in serotonin, and this increase in serotonin elevates mood. This is the same thing that happens with many of the antidepressant drugs on the market; serotonin levels are elevated and the person feels better.

High fiber foods are complex carbohydrates. Fiber provides bulk in the diet. Bulk in the diet helps with the feeling of satiety. Fiber foods have greater volume and slow gastric emptying, which is a signal for the body to stop eating. Fiber requires more chewing, which slows the rate and increases the effort it takes to consume food. This also gives the body the signal of being full. High fiber foods are also more satisfying because they carry nutrients further down into the small intestine. Research shows that these feelings of satiety from complex carbs and fiber may last up to twelve to fourteen hours after eating. So it can be said that fiber affects the amount of food ingested by exerting a suppressive effect on a person's feelings of hunger.

There are several high protein diets, which are popular at this time. You will lose weight on a high protein diet! Garanteed! But before you start one of these high protein diets, you should be aware of some of the potential adverse effects. If you still choose to go on a high protein diet, make sure you have decided the benefits outweigh the risks.

Almost everything eaten on a high protein diet is protein. Protein foods are mostly meat, cheese, and dairy products. These foods are high in calories and saturated fat. There are no or very few carbohydrates on a true high protein diet. So how does this make you lose weight?

High protein diets change how your body metabolizes food. Carbohydrates are so severely limited that lean body tissue, as well as fat, is broken down for fuel. This causes a condition called ketosis. You lose weight because of the process of ketosis. Usually this is not a problem for a short period of time as your body makes adjustments for the ketosis. But if you are on a high protein diet for an extended period of time or if you have kidney problems, you may develop some serious health problems.

How do you know if your body is in a ketoic state? Test a urine sample with a urine dipstick, the kind found in any health clinic. If your body is in a ketoic state, the dipstick will show that you have ketones in your urine. I know people who have been on high protein diets that check their urine regularly to see if they have reached a ketoic state.

Problems that can be encountered on a high protein diet include heart and kidney diseases. Since proteins contain saturated fats, if you stay on a high protein diet for an extended period of time, you risk developing health problems associated with high fat diets, including cardiovascular disease, heart attacks, and strokes.

The kidneys have to work extra hard to eliminate the byproducts of protein metabolism. Over time, this can cause renal insuffiency and failure or other kidney problems. If you have ketones and protein in your urine consistently, your kidneys are working overtime.

Excess protein can also cause calcium deficiencies and jeopardize the health of your bones. With a large protein intake, calcium is lost from the bones and excreted in the urine. Loss of calcium leads to osteoporosis, which leads to the risk of hip and other fractures. This applies equally to men and women.

There is increased risk of liver damage with high protein diets. The liver must work harder to metabolize the protein, similar to what happens with the kidneys.

In high protein diets, there is an increase in the amount of uric acid in the body. This leads to an increased risk of developing gout (painful inflammation of joints caused by uric acid crystals lodging in the joint). Treatment consists of eliminating the foods that are causing the gout and anti-inflammatory pain medication. Foods that contribute to the development of gout are foods high in purines such as anchovies, beer, sardines, yeast, and organ meats such as liver and kidney.

Another diet is the Formula diet meaning one or more meals is replaced with a liquid formula, usually some type of protein drink. These are easy to use for short term weight loss but are not effective long term. One drawback is the fact these diets are not usually balanced diets. You cannot get all the vitamins, minerals, and fiber you need in your diet with liquid supplements. Neither do these diets teach you how to make healthy food choices. Therefore, most people regain the weight as soon as they stop using the products and have to make their own food choices. These diets are difficult to maintain for an extended period of time as drinking your food does not give you the feelings of satiety that you get from chewing your food.

Many diet programs promote special or prepackaged foods. You buy your food from these companies, and this is a large portion or all of what you eat while you lose weight. These diets have been designed to give you a balanced diet that is low in calories and fat. Again, the problem is, once you lose the weight and go back to eating "everyday food" you gain the weight back. For permanent weight loss you are going to have to learn to make choices for a balanced diet using the foods that are in your own world and eat these in the proper proportions to your caloric needs.

Similar to the special foods diet is the "fixed menu" diet. These are the ones you see in magazines, where you are given a menu for every day for a certain amount of time along with the shopping list for foods on the menu. These are usually easy to follow, but there are only a few food choices, which lead to boredom in a short period of time, making the diet hard to stick to. There is also no allowance for eating out on these diets, and you aren't learning any food selection skills with these.

Last, there are "exchange type" diets. With these diets you may choose foods from all food groups. There is usually a point system or other way to determine the amount of food you are allowed to eat. These diets are easily followed away from home, and you learn food selection skills. They are probably the closest you are going to come to a perfect diet.

So what is the "perfect diet?" The perfect diet should be individualized for each person. It means choosing the right amount of carbs, fats, proteins, and calories that creates weight loss now and weight maintenance in the future. Your optimal weight must also be individualized for you. Your ideal weight needs to be a healthy weight where you look and feel your best. That is what you are going to learn to do in the next chapters.

Discontent is the first step in the progress of a man or a nation.

Chapter Five

Making Choices

So far, you've learned about the problem we face in the country regarding obesity. You've had a brief overview of how the digestive process works and about the many hormones and other factors that affect our weight. Next, you are going to learn your role in all this and what you can do to lose the weight you want and need to lose and how you can maintain this weight loss for life.

One fundamental concept that you must learn in order to lose weight and maintain your weight loss has to do with choices. You may often feel the external world controls you and your choices are based on these external controls. However, you are much more in control of your life and your choices than you may realize. Other people cannot make your choices for you. They can't make you sad or happy. They can't force you to put food in your mouth. You choose everything you do. I doubt if anyone has ever put a gun to your head and said, "Eat!"

You are in control of your choices, but, unfortunately, much of that control may be ineffective, especially when it comes to what you eat. By learning to take more effective control of your actions and eating habits and patterns you will learn to make more effective choices. The wrong choices destroy happiness and health. The right choices will give you happiness, health, and longevity.

There are two types of control in your life, internal control and external control. How are they different? External control is an attempt to control someone else's behavior or situation, and there are people who will try to control your behavior when it comes to eating. Perhaps you have already experienced this. Internal control is when you make the decisions that affect your life. Internal control puts you in charge of your behavior and situation.

Someone once told me, "Everything is your own fault. If it isn't, you can't do anything about it." I think by this they meant I had to take responsibility for the things that happened to me. Only then could I change things and make things happen the way I wanted them to. I had to learn to use internal control.

Let's examine external control more closely. William Glasser, in his book on Choice Theory (1998), gave three beliefs about external control. He said first, you are responding to something. For example, stopping at a stop light. The light turns red, and you respond by stopping. Second, you can control other people and what they do OR other people can control you and what you do. Third, rewards and punishments are used to control others. Some words used to describe external control are coerce, force, compel, manipulate, boss, antagonize, blame, complain, nag, badger, etc.

Glasser goes on to explain how external control is used by much of the world. With external control you are the victim, you have no self-control. With internal control on the other hand, you make your own choices from within yourself. For example, you are reading this book. You are taking in the information that is written in this book. The information you gain from the book can't make you do anything. You can choose to act on it or ignore it. If you decide to use the information, you have chosen to use it based on the information you have been given. You make a decision, you choose to use it. You won't lose weight by just reading this book. You have to choose to use the information that is given to you.

By practicing internal control you cannot blame others for your situation. As I said earlier, if something isn't your fault, you can't do anything about it. But by choosing an action, the result of that action is your fault, and you are the one who can change the result or do something about that result because it is your choice.

By practicing internal control you do not control others, only yourself and your actions. You recognize that they too are responsible for their own actions. Your own actions are the only thing you can do anything about. Their actions are the only thing they can do anything about.

As you learn to apply this concept of internal control to losing weight, try applying it to other areas of your life also. Not only will your weight and health improve, but all your interactions with other people will improve.

As you go through life, you learn to surround yourself with people and things that help you satisfy your needs. Glasser calls this your "quality world." It is built on your perception of how you interpret information you receive. What you choose to put in your quality world makes you feel good and satisfies your wants in life. Food and eating are two things you put in your quality world.

Food is part of almost everyone's quality world. The exception would be a person who is an anorexic and has chosen to take food out of their quality world. Right now the foods you eat and your lifestyle are the ones you have chosen to put in your quality world. You are continually creating and recreating your quality world through the choices you make. The purpose of this book is to teach you to recreate your quality world in relation to the foods you eat and the lifestyle you choose. You will learn to make more effective choices, so you can practice internal control rather than external control.

Your actions are your behavior. You attempt to adjust your actions, or your behavior, to gain control over your life. Behavior is either effective or ineffective. Effective behavior means you are behaving or acting in such a way that you are satisfying your needs in your quality world. Your choices should be helping you to do this. You feel good when you are doing something that gives you effective control in your life. As you make, implement, and see results from the weight loss plan you develop, you are going to feel good because you will be demonstrating that you have control over your life, your behavior, and your actions.

When you change your behavior, you can change what you want, what you are doing, or both. You probably have a good idea of what you want right now, so my job is to help you change what you are doing. In the end, you may find you have made a change in both. Sometimes what you think you want is modified as you make progress towards your goals.

Remember, it is your quality world and not anyone or anything can prevent you from making your own choices. Dr. Robert Wubbolding, who has worked with Dr. Glasser for many years, says the choices you make will determine the life you lead. How very true.

You now know that behavior is a choice. Behavior consists of your actions, thinking, feelings, and your physiology (your body). You choose your actions, choose what you think, and choose what you feel. By making effective choices, you affect the physiology of your body (how you look and feel).

You are going to learn to take total control of your actions and thoughts, and by taking total control of your actions and thoughts you will take total control of your life. If you make a choice that turns out not to be as good a choice as you had hoped, you can choose to make a better choice next time. For example, if you go out to eat at a restaurant and you order food you think is low calorie or low fat and it turns out not to be, next time you eat at that particular restaurant don't order that food again or ask to have it modified if possible.

Choices are generally not reversible. Once you make a choice and carry through with it, you are responsible for the consequences. If you eat a dessert with one thousand calories and gain weight from this, you are responsible for the weight gain, no one else is. No one forced you to choose that dessert and made you eat it. Remember, you choose what you do, but you are capable of choosing something better. You could have chosen a dessert with fewer calories and more food value. If it is a choice, you are responsible for making that choice, and you are responsible for the consequences.

Learning to make better choices leads to optimism and a positive attitude. You will feel freer, happier, and will have more control over your life. Pessimism comes from feeling a situation is hopeless and you can't do anything about it. Remember, everything is your fault, or you can't do anything about it.

When you accept that your chosen thoughts and actions may have a great deal to do with your weight and your health, you have already begun to change your quality world and the physiology of your body. Changing what you think and your attitude has a major impact on your life.

Some people need and choose to work with their health care providers to use medicine and/or surgery to help decrease their weight. In some instances this is medically necessary. In those instances these may be appropriate choices to make. You and your health care provider are the ones who must decide if this needs to be part of your weight loss program. You are the one who has to make the final choice on what you will do. If you choose this as part of your program just remember that the medicine and/or the surgery isn't going to solve the whole problem. You will have to make the choice and learn how to change your eating habits and your lifestyle. These are the choices that will determine if you maintain the weight loss for life. If you choose medicine and/or surgery and don't make appropriate lifestyle changes, you will regain the weight you lose.

Making healthy choices does not always come easy in a culture like ours of external control. You can't blame the fast food restaurants or others for making you overweight. You must take control of your life and not let these outside influences control your life. It may be hard. It may be a challenge. It may be the most difficult thing you have ever done in your life. But deciding to make your own choices will definitely lead to a healthier, happier life for you. Learning to take internal control and make your own choices on food and lifestyle will eventually carry over to other areas of your life and give you control and freedom you never knew existed.

The choices you make will determine the life you lead.
-Robert Wubbolding

Chapter Six

Putting Choices into Action

In the last chapter, we talked about choices. Your first choice is to make the decision to lose weight. Your body is your most valuable asset and possession. Yes, your body is a possession. It is yours to do with as you see fit. It is your most valuable possession because you can't do anything in life without your body. How well you take care of your body will be one of the factors that will determine other things you can do in life. Being overweight or obese limits the number of physical things you can do and how well you can do them. Being overweight or obese also puts you at risk for many, many diseases and adverse health conditions. Being overweight or obese has an impact on how you make a living and how well you will live.

Along with your choice to lose weight is the realization that there are things you will have to give up and lifestyle changes you will have to make. You may have to give up some of your friends if they are preventing you from reaching your goal to lose weight. You may have to give up, change or modify some of your social situations. Some of these lifestyle changes may not be easy. At times, you will have to make a choice between immediate gratification and reaching your long term goal.

Ask yourself the following questions. Am I willing to change my lifestyle permanently to achieve my weight loss goals? Am I willing to eat differently than my family or friends even though it may cause conflict? Am I ready to face the possibility of having to give up friends who do not support me or will sabotage my efforts to lose weight? Am I willing to do what it takes to achieve my goals? Am I ready to accept the idea that I am the only person responsible for the choices I make and the only one who can do anything about what happens in my life. Your willpower will be tested, but you have to remember, when you look in the mirror every morning, you are looking at the only person who is responsible for achieving your weight loss and other goals in your life. Remember the old saying, "If it is to be, it's up to me."

It is now time to get started. To develop your plan you are first going to have to obtain some baseline information about yourself. Even though losing weight may seem like a simple thing to do, it may be a major change for your body. The first thing you want to do is make sure you do not have any health issues you are unaware of. Some health conditions must be addressed prior to beginning a weight loss program. See your health care provider prior to starting your weight loss program to make sure you do not have a health condition that would interfere with your progress or the changes you want to make.

Make an appointment to see your health care provider for a general physical exam. The physical exam should include: a review of your current health problems and medications, blood pressure and heart rate, screening lab that includes a fasting lipid profile, fasting blood sugar, and TSH (thyroid stimulating hormone).

The fasting lipid profile should include your total cholesterol, LDL (low density lipoprotein or bad cholesterol), HDL (high density lipoprotein or good cholesterol), and triglycerides. The fasting blood sugar is to screen for Diabetes and the TSH to screen for Hypothyroidism, which can affect your metabolism and prevent you from loosing weight.

Cholesterol got you confused? HDL cholesterol is considered to be good cholesterol. The HDL, or good cholesterol, carries cholesterol to the liver, where it is excreted from the body. The best way to increase your HDL is with exercise. LDL cholesterol is considered to be bad cholesterol. The LDL, or bad cholesterol, allows cholesterol to accumulate in the bloodstream, where it lodges on the blood vessel walls as plaque. Plaque can either occlude the blood vessel or can break loose and travel through the blood as a thrombi (clot), causing a heart attack or stroke. These are things you are trying to prevent. Your diet has a direct effect on your LDL. Genetics (your genes) affect both HDL and LDL and is something you cannot change.

If your fasting lipid profile is abnormal, your health care provider may want you to go on a low cholesterol diet or take medication to bring the abnormal levels back to normal. So being there to see your provider because you are wanting to start a healthy living program will be just the thing they want you to do.

If you are over forty years old, have high blood pressure, an abnormally slow, rapid or irregular heart rate, have a heart murmur, or have a family history of heart disease or stroke, especially in relatives less than sixty years old, your health care provider many want you to have an EKG and/or exercise stress test to screen for heart disease or other cardiac abnormalities.

Hopefully, you won't ignore this part of your program. An example of why this is an important first step can be illustrated with a story about a friend of mine. This friend had started getting short-of-breath when he was in his forties. He was a little overweight, so he decided the shortness of breath was due to being overweight and out-of-shape. He embarked on a "diet" and exercise program that included running. The weight came off, and he thought he was getting healthier; however, the shortness of breath did not get better. Finally, he went to see his health care provider and was diagnosed with lung cancer. He died six months later. Perhaps if he had had a physical exam prior to his weight loss program, the outcome would have been better or at least maybe he would have lived longer than six months.

So be smart. Make sure you are healthy and don't have any preexisting conditions that would prevent or interfere with your lifestyle modification and exercise plan. You don't want complications to develop along the way, and if you have a condition that might prevent you from accomplishing your weight loss goals, why not find out at the beginning and do something about it. It will be easier to reach your goals if you don't have obstacles in your way.

While you are with your health care provider, discuss what a realistic goal weight should be for you. Also, get their input on any special health conditions you have that might affect what you want your weight to be.

After you have obtained your medical clearance, you will want to do a self-assessment. I recommend you purchase or make some type of notebook, where you can write this information down. You are going to want to have your plan on paper and not just in your head. Many people don't want to "go to this much trouble" to lose weight, but trust me, you have to have an accurate idea of where you are starting from to plan where you want to go.

First, you want to find out what your initial weight is. I recommend you weigh yourself first thing in the morning after going to the bathroom. Either weigh in your underwear or in the nude. If it is not convenient to weigh yourself first thing in the morning, then weigh yourself at the same time of day, wearing the same clothing and after going to the bathroom. What you are wearing and having a full bladder can make a difference of as much as several pounds in your weight. You may think you have lost or not lost weight when it may only be a reflection of HOW you are weighing yourself.

When you weigh yourself you are weighing bones, muscle, fat, and fluid. The weight gain or loss you see on the scale can be water weight, fat weight, or muscle weight. An understanding of how these fluctuate will help keep you from becoming frustrated from lack of results some weeks or erratic fluctuations in your weight. Frustration and lack of weight loss is what causes some people to give up on their weight loss goals.

Water weight refers to the weight of all the water in your body. This weight is found in your bloodstream, the cells and tissues in your body and in your digestive tract. It varies daily, depending on how well-hydrated or dehydrated you are.

Fat weight refers to the weight of all the fat in your body. This includes the fat on your abdomen, thighs, arms, and other areas you want to lose weight. There is also fat in and around your organs and all cells of your body. This fat is essential for life. Fat contains very little water.

Fat is important in the body. It protects your internal organs, insulates your body from the cold, and is an important source of stored vitamins and minerals. It functions as your primary source of stored energy. Because of these important functions of fat if you begin to lose weight too rapidly, your body will automatically trigger mechanisms to slow this weight loss down to protect you. This is sometimes what is happening when you reach a plateau. Once your body has adjusted to the changes you are making, you will start to lose weight again. If this happens, just be patient and continue what you are doing.

Muscle weight is lean weight. The loss of muscle weight is something you DON'T want to happen. When you lose muscle weight, your metabolism decreases. The loss of muscle weight occurs when you have a sedentary lifestyle, when you take in too few calories (a very low calorie diet) and is part of the aging process. Muscle weight loss can be prevented by increased activity and a regular exercise program. This is one important reason to remain active and continue to exercise regularly as you grow older. Muscles weigh more than fat. But that is a good thing. Muscle weight is the type of weight you DO want.

Weight can also be lost from bone. When this occurs a person has a condition called osteoporosis and should be diagnosed and treated by a health care provider. The loss of bone weight can be slowed or prevented with a diet high in calcium and vitamin D along with a regular exercise program. This is one reason you need to maintain a balanced diet while losing weight. If your body does not get the vitamins and minerals it needs to function properly, it WILL take these vitamins and minerals from somewhere else in the body in order to function properly. An example is calcium. You must have a certain level of calcium in your bloodstream to meet the body's daily needs for this mineral (for example, for your heart to function properly). If you do not have normal levels of calcium in the bloodstream, it will be taken from the bones and used. If this happens over a period of time, such as when a person is trying to lose weight, then osteoporosis will develop.

When you talk about losing weight, you are really talking about losing fat weight. The gain and loss of fat is continually occurring in the body. Your body has a certain amount of energy it needs daily. When your total energy requirement exceeds your total energy consumed, you loose fat weight. When you consume more energy than you use, you gain fat weight. This is expressed by the term "calories." So when you use more calories than you consume, you lose fat weight. When you consume more calories than you use, you gain fat weight. When the number of calories you consume equals the number of calories you burn, your weight stays the same.

When you start to lose weight, you will see fluctuations in your weight. Don't become frustrated. Just continue to do what you are doing, but note the patterns of your weight gain or loss. After a period of time, you will begin to know your weight loss patterns and can determine whether the gain or loss is related to fat loss, water loss, muscle loss, or a combination of these.

You will want to plan to weigh yourself at least weekly. Some people prefer to weigh daily. Either one is acceptable (although some books insist on one or the other) as long as you are consistent in what you do. I wouldn't go longer than a week without weighing as this can be discouraging if you don't show much loss. I will show you how to plot this on a graph, so you will actually be able to see your results over time (see Appendix).

There are several ways to determine what would be a good weight range for you. One is the use of a BMI chart. BMI stands for Body Mass Index. BMI is a ratio that indicates whether your weight is appropriate for your height. It reflects body fat in most adults. You can determine your BMI by looking at your current height and weight on the BMI chart provided in the Appendix.

A BMI less than 18.5 is considered underweight, 18.5 to 24.9 is normal, and 25 to 30 is overweight. A BMI greater than thirty is considered obese. The BMI chart is not accurate for very fit people who weigh more because they are muscular or for children and teenagers.

Another method some people use to determine approximately what they should weigh goes like this. For women, you should weigh 100 pounds for the first 5 feet and 5 pounds for each additional inch over 5 feet. For men it is 110 pounds for the first 5 feet and 10 pounds for each additional inch over 5 feet. An example of this would be a woman 5 ft. 4 in. tall should weigh 120 pounds. A man 5 ft. 10 in. tall should weigh 160 pounds. There are also many Ideal Body Weight Charts that have been published. If you use one of these just make sure it is from a reliable source.

Use the BMI chart or other method to determine your goal weight as a guide. You want to reach a weight where you feel good and are healthy. As you lose weight, you will find where this weight is. If you reach a weight where you feel good and are healthy but your BMI is higher than 25, discuss this with your health care provider. This may be the ideal weight for you. Statistics and charts can't dictate the weight you feel good at and are healthy at.

If you have a lot of weight to lose, you don't want to think about the entire amount at one time. It might seem overwhelming that you could lose a large amount of weight. Use a range for the weight you want to lose. For example, if you need and want to lose one hundred pounds, focus on short term goals of ten or fifteen pounds. Once you lose this ten or fifteen pounds, focus on the next ten or fifteen pounds. Another technique is to focus on one month at a time. Make a goal of losing five or ten pounds a month (or one to two pounds per week). Remember that the weight you lose slowly is the weight you are more likely to keep off.

Some people use their initial weight loss goal as 10% of their weight. For example, if you weigh 200 pounds, your initial weight loss goal might be 20 pounds or a goal weight of 180 pounds. Once reaching 180 pounds, the next goal would be to lose 18 pounds or a goal weight of 162 pounds. If the final goal weight is lower than 162 pounds, you would keep going with the same pattern. It is much easier and less overwhelming to have a weight loss goal of 20 pounds instead of say 100 pounds.

Along with recording of your initial weight, you will want to record your height. Everyone should have their height checked yearly, not just growing children. Having your height checked yearly can be your first clue to the development of osteoporosis or other abnormal bone conditions if you are losing height. Also record waist, hip and bust measurements, upper and midthighs, upper arms and calves. There is a chart in the Appendix that you can copy and use for this purpose. Take these measurements weekly or monthly, your choice. You will know when these measurements are changing as you will begin to notice a difference in how your clothes fit – they will be getting looser.

Next, on your way to starting your weight loss program, I want you to write down in your notebook all the things you have done in the past to lose weight. You might use two pages for this. On one page, write down the things that did not work and WHY. On the other page, write down the things that helped you lose weight and keep it off and WHY. We will use this information later when you start to make your new plan. The things that didn't work before are things you are going to avoid this time.

And last, in your preparation for your new weight loss program, I want you to keep a food diary for one to two weeks. Don't change your eating habits at all during this time. Write down what you eat, how much, when, the location of where you are eating, your activity at the time and your feelings and thoughts associated with eating at that time. Again, there is a chart in the Appendix that you can use as a guide for this. Also included will be the number of calories.

All this information will give you baseline information for starting your weight loss program. This may seem like a lot of trouble because I know you just want to "get started and lose weight," but it is difficult to determine where you want to go and be successful if you don't know and understand where you are starting from and what you have done in the past. It is difficult to reach a goal without a plan, and your baseline information is part of your plan.

Remember your body is your most valuable asset and possession. You are in the process of learning more about your most valuable asset and how to take better care of it. Think of the book you are creating when you are writing information down as you do the owner's manual to your car. All the specifics you need to know to take the best care of your body will be in this book. It will serve as a guide for you in taking care of your body much as the owner's manual is a guide for taking care of your car.

*It's the moment you think you can't that you
realize you can.*

Chapter Seven

Food and Water Basics

One thing that many people do when they start a weight loss program is to radically change what or how they eat. This may involve severely limiting the quantity and amount of their food choices. When this is done, the person not only deprives themselves of foods they enjoy, but their diet may be lacking in vitamins and minerals essential for their health. The person can usually do this for awhile but then fails at their attempt to lose weight because they cannot continue with the eating pattern they have established.

To lose weight successfully and maintain your weight loss you must develop eating habits you can continue for the rest of your life. Most people don't have to radically change what or how they eat, but there are some basic guidelines for a well-balanced diet that need to be followed. It is important to have balance and variety in what you eat, but to eat in moderation. You may have to learn to think differently and make different choices about the food you eat. You want to learn to make healthy food choices while gradually eliminating unhealthy food choices. Your timetable for this will be established when you develop your goals.

Your body needs a variety of vitamins, minerals, and other food substances to remain healthy. In general, you should have 2 to 3 servings of protein, 2 to 3 servings of dairy products, 2 to 3 servings of fruit, 4 to 6 servings of vegetables, and 5 to 6 servings of whole grains daily. You will know if you are getting these recommended servings as you keep and evaluate your food diary.

Let's talk about the Food Diary for a minute. Remember that studies show if you keep a food diary, you will be more successful in your weight management program over time. In your Food Diary, you need to keep a record of everything you eat for one or two weeks. When I say "everything," I do mean "everything." Often, those little "snacks" or "munchies" or "just a taste" of things will add up to several hundred calories by the end of a day. These are the things that may make the difference between being successful and not successful in your weight management program. At the end of the two weeks, you are going to analyze your food intake to determine where you can realistically make changes. You may be surprised where extra calories are coming from. You may also discover where you can eliminate extra calories and never miss them. You only have to eliminate five hundred to one thousand calories per day to lose one to two pounds per week. You can also look at this another way. You only have to use or burn an additional five hundred or one thousand calories per day to lose one or two pounds per week.

So where do you find out the number of calories and other nutritional info about food? Many foods now have some type of nutritional label on the package. I encourage you to start reading these labels and become familiar with the number of calories the foods you usually eat contain as well as the other nutritional information written on the label.

Nutrition Facts

Serving Size 2 crackers (14 g)
Servings Per Container About 21

Amount Per Serving

Calories 60   Calories from Fat 15

	% Daily Value*
Total Fat 1.5g	2%
Saturated Fat 0g	0%
Trans Fat 0g	
Cholesterol 0mg	0%
Sodium 70mg	3%
Total Carbohydrate 10g	3%
Dietary Fiber Less than 1g	3%
Sugars 0g	
Protein 2g	

Vitamin A 0%   •   Vitamin C 0%

Calcium 0%   •   Iron 2%

* Percent Daily Values are based on a 2,000 calorie diet. Your daily values may be higher or lower depending on your calorie needs:

		Calories:	2,000	2,500
Total Fat	Less than		65g	80g
Sat Fat	Less than		20g	25g
Cholesterol	Less than		300mg	300mg
Sodium	Less than		2400mg	2400mg
Total Carbohydrate			300g	375g
Dietary Fiber			25g	30g

To read a food label you first need to know what some of the abbreviations mean. Vitamins, minerals, and other nutrients are measured in grams (g) or milligrams (mg). Some of the information will be listed as a percentage (%). The values given are the amount in one serving and based on a diet where you consume two thousand calories per day.

Look at the nutrition label shown. It comes from a box of snack crackers. Below the words Nutrition Facts, you will find the serving size which in this case is two crackers. There are about twenty-one servings per box. Next is listed the number of calories per serving or the number of calories that two crackers contain. In this case two crackers contain sixty calories. To find the number of calories per cracker divide two into sixty. Each cracker will have thirty calories.

Calories tell you have much energy is in food. A calorie is a unit of measurement or a unit of energy. Your body has to have calories for energy. Food and liquids contain calories. Calories are described in grams (gm) on the food label. Carbohydrates, protein, fiber, fat, alcohol, and water contain a certain number of calories per gram (gm).

1 gm of carbohydrate = 4 calories
1 gm of protein = 4 calories
1 gm of fiber = 2 calories
1 gm of fat = 9 calories
1 gm of alcohol = 7 calories
1 gm of water = 0 calories

If you are concerned about the amount of fat in your diet, you want to look at the calories from fat on the food label, which is usually across from the calories per serving. Notice that fat contains more than twice the number of calories per gram as some of the other food nutrients at nine calories per gram.

Next on the food label, the percent daily value is listed. These percentages are based on recommended daily allowances or the amount of the nutrient a person should get in the diet each day. For example, on the food label below, the amount of sodium in a serving of crackers is 70mg which is 3% of the recommended daily allowance for an adult. Notice that these crackers contain 0gms of saturated and trans fat, which is good as the recommended daily allowance for these is 0%.

Some of the percent daily values are based on the number of calories and amount of energy a person needs, which includes carbohydrates, proteins, and fat. The percent daily values for vitamins and minerals stay the same no matter how many calories a person eats.

The total fat on the food label is the number of fat grams contained in one serving of the crackers. Fat is an essential food element. Unsaturated fat is the fat that is good in your diet. You want to avoid the saturated and trans fats. Notice these are all listed separately on the label.

Sodium and cholesterol are included on food labels. These numbers tell you how much sodium (salt) and cholesterol are in a single serving of the food. These are included because some people need to limit the amount of salt in their diet (for example, people with high blood pressure or heart problems) or the amount of cholesterol in their diet (people with high cholesterol).

Many foods on the market are labeled as "low fat," "low sodium," etc. This can be very confusing. The information below will serve as a guide to help you understand what these terms mean.

Calorie free: Less than 5 calories per serving.

Sugar free: less than 0.5 gm of sugar per serving.

Fat free: less than 0.5 gm of fat per serving.

Low fat: 3 gm of fat or less per serving.

Reduced fat or less fat: 25% less fat than the regular product.

Low in saturated fat: 1 gm of saturated fat or less, with not more than 15% of the calories coming from saturated fat per serving.

Lean: less than 10 gm of fat, 4 gm of saturated fat and 95 mg of cholesterol per serving.

Extra lean: less than 5 gm of fat, 2 gm of saturated fat, and 95 mg of cholesterol per serving.

Light (lite): at least one-third fewer calories, or no more than half the fat of the regular product, or no more than half the sodium of the regular product per serving.

Cholesterol free: less than 2 mg of cholesterol and 2 gm (or less) of saturated fat per serving.

Low cholesterol: 20 or fewer mg of cholesterol and 2 gm or less of saturated fat per serving.

Reduced cholesterol: at least 25% less cholesterol than the regular product and 2 gm or less of saturated fat per serving.

Sodium free or no sodium: less than 5 mg of sodium and no sodium chloride in ingredients per serving.

Very low sodium: 35 mg or less of sodium per serving.

Low sodium: 140 mg or less of sodium per serving.

Reduced or less sodium: 25% less sodium than the regular product per serving.

High fiber: 5 gm or more of fiber per serving.

Good source of fiber: 2.5 to 4.9 gm of fiber per serving.

Not all foods have food labels. The foods that are outrageously high in calories and fat don't always have nutritional labels. Neither do your very nutritious foods have food labels. When you go to a grocery store and purchase fresh fruits and vegetables, you will seldom see a food label unless they are prepackaged. Food from restaurants seldom has nutritional info, although it may be available if you ask for it. My suggestion is that you purchase a good food count book that gives you the nutritional information about foods you buy in the grocery store as well as the nutritional information about food from the most popular franchise restaurants. There are many of these on the market today. Find one you like and one that has information on food from restaurants you frequently eat at. You aren't going to want to stop eating at your favorite restaurants, so you are going to need to learn how to make better food choices at these restaurants. If the restaurants you eat at aren't listed in any book you find, ask at the restaurant for the nutritional information on the food they serve.

You may have heard the terms "low energy dense food" or "high energy dense food." This is one very important component of food that is missing from food labels. It is a component which you will have to figure yourself but is easy to do. Energy density (E.D.) refers to is the caloric density of the food or the calories per gram. A "low energy dense food" has a low number of calories per gram, whereas a "high energy dense food" has a larger number of calories per gram. In simple terms, this means that you can eat a large volume of food when you are eating low energy dense foods.

An example of a low energy dense food is a serving of green beans. The food label on a can of green beans says that a serving is ½ cup and has 20 calories or 120 gm per serving. To find the E.D. of the green beans divide 20 calories by 120 gm. The E.D. for green beans is .16. So we can say the green beans have a very low energy density. Compare this to the snack crackers in our food label example above. Divide the 60 calories by 14 gm, and the E.D. of the crackers is 4.3, which makes the crackers a high energy dense food. This tells you that you can eat a much larger volume of the green beans than you can the crackers and have a lower caloric intake.

Some books divide energy density into categories. These categories are Very Low Energy Dense foods (0 to 0.6), Low Energy Dense foods (0.6 to 1.5), Medium Energy Dense foods (1.5 to 1.4), and High Energy Dense foods (4.0 to 9.0). Along with calories use E.D. to help guide you in your food choices.

You won't always have a calculator with you to figure E.D. Use these guidelines as a rule of thumb for E.D. If the calories in the food are lower than the number of grams, eat what you want (within reason). If the calories in the food are the same or up to twice as many as the grams in the food, use portion control. If the calories in the food are more than twice the number of grams in the food, eat only a small portion of the food or consider not eating the food at all.

Along with the basic food groups and number of servings you should try to eat daily is your daily intake of water. Your daily intake of water should be eight or nine 8 oz. glasses every twenty-four hours. Out of all the vitamins, minerals, and nutrients that your body needs, water is the most essential. Your body functions better when you are well hydrated. If your body is not well hydrated, almost all the functions of your body are compromised, including your metabolism.

More than half of your body weight is water weight, 60 to 70% to be more exact. Water is lost daily through the digestive process but also from perspiration, respiration, and many other bodily functions. Water is used in many of the chemical reactions that occur when you are burning calories whether at rest or with activity. When you don't get enough water, or you become dehydrated, the digestive process is compromised and you may not get all the vitamins and minerals that have been consumed with your food. Dehydration may trigger some of those hormonal reactions discussed earlier, telling you to eat more food. When you are dehydrated, your body may think it is hungry when all it really needs is water.

There are other benefits to water. You can use water to make your body think it is more full than it is. You will be given several strategies for this when you start to develop your plan, but for right now I'm just going to say that by drinking enough water you can curb your appetite. Water can be used to fill you up, and it can be used to dilute certain foods so that you are eating a larger food volume with fewer calories.

When you exercise, you burn calories, but you also lose water through increased metabolic demands such as increased perspiration and increased respiratory rates. Your body will be using water that is already stored, and when this is gone, it must be replaced. Additional water is needed to cool your body as your body temperature increases with exercise. As you exercise more, you will replace fat with lean muscle tissue and muscle tissue needs and holds much more water than fat tissue does.

Drinks such as coffee, tea, and soda pop are not a substitute for water even though they contain water. All of these contain a certain amount of caffeine which acts as a diuretic, which can actually have a dehydrating effect on your body. Soda pop contains phosphoric acid, which, if consumed in large enough quantities, can stimulate the loss of calcium for bones contributing to osteoporosis.

Tips for increasing water in your diet include carrying a bottle of water with you to be sipped on throughout the day. Use soda pop and other beverages as rewards for drinking water first. For example, you might allow yourself one small soda pop after you have consumed your eight glasses of water for the day. Substitute herbal teas for the regular tea or coffee. Herbal teas generally do not contain caffeine. Have a glass of water before meals and drink water between bites when eating your meals. Not only does this help keep you hydrated, but the water before and during the meal will help you fill fuller sooner and you will eat less at the meal.

You deserve to be healthy.

You deserve to be a healthy weight.

The Samurai: From the moment they wake they devote themselves to perfecting that which they have chosen.

Chapter Eight

Creating Your Plan

I am going to teach you to make a plan, the framework of which comes from "Choice Theory," developed by Dr. William Glasser and expanded on by Dr. Robert Wubbolding, using "Reality Therapy." It is based on answering the questions, What do you want and what are you doing now? It includes self-evaluation and making your plan. This is called the WDEP approach.

> W: "What do you want?"
> D: "What are you doing?"
> E: "Evaluation"
> P: "Plan"

What do you want?

Back to your paper and pen. Take a sheet of paper. Write down how much weight you want and need to lose. In addition to the answers to how much weight you want and need to lose, write down all the reasons it is important to you to lose weight. If losing weight and being healthy are important to you, then these are considered to be your values. Your values are part of what we will call your "quality world." If you want to lose weight only for reasons that are important to other people, then stop right here—losing weight will never be one of your values and part of your "quality world." Losing weight has to be something, you want for yourself.

Let me give you an example. If you want to lose weight so you will be healthier, look better, and feel better, these are reasons that matter to you, that you value. If you want to lose weight because someone else in your life wants you to and you would only be doing it for them it isn't going to work. You may lose some weight and keep it off for a period of time, but if it isn't something you want and value, then you will never keep the weight off for any length of time.

What are you doing now?

Write down what you are currently doing to lose weight AND how you feel about what you are currently doing to lose weight. How you feel about what you are doing will have an impact on how successful you are. If you feel good about what you are doing, it is easier to keep doing it. On the other hand, if you don't have good feelings about what you are doing, you probably will not continue the action for very long. What you don't feel good about doing is not and probably never will be one of your values and will never become part of your quality world. Feelings have a big impact on your actions. You have to feel good about something for it to work for you.

Evaluation:

Take the information from Chapter Six where you wrote down and evaluated what you had done in the past to lose weight and why or why it didn't work. Add to that the information you have about what you are currently doing. Is what you are currently doing to lose weight working, why or why not? Are the things you are currently doing, or things you did in the past to lose weight, changes you could permanently incorporate into your eating habits and lifestyle? Will you achieve your weight loss and health goals if you continue this behavior? Write down each thing you are currently doing or have done in the past and answer yes or no beside of it. Evaluating what you have done and what you are currently doing will help you make changes that will help you be more successful in the future.

Plan:

After you evaluate what you have done in the past and are currently doing, you are ready to make your plan. Your plan is going to be a realistic, workable, flexible plan to lose weight, designed specifically for you.

The components of your plan can be described with the acronym: SAMICC. Your plan will be:

S : Simple
A : Attainable
M: Measurable
I : Immediate, with your involvement
C : Controlled by you
C : Consistent and committed to by you

You actually have already started your plan with your baseline information from Chapter Six. So far you have seen or made an appointment with your health care provider for a physical exam and to discuss your plan to start a weight loss and management program, and had or will have, any tests or further testing recommended by your provider. You have determined a realistic goal weight to work towards, recorded your current height and weight and other measurements discussed, listed things you have done in the past and are currently doing to manage your weight, evaluated these, and have started keeping a food diary. You are off to a great start! Good job!!

You now have enough information to determine your goals and create your weight loss and management plan.

<u>Making Your Plan and Setting Your goals</u>

There are four basic guidelines to follow when setting goals. They are:

1. Your goals must be specific and measurable.
2. To reach your goals you must be willing to do what it takes to achieve your goals.
3. You need to make both short term goals (STGs) and long term goals (LTGs).
4. Work toward your STGs to accomplish your LTGs.

So let's make your goals! As you make your goals, remember to make goals that will make you happy.

Make big goals! Shoot for the stars, even if you only reach the moon, you will be able to look at how far you have traveled. Big goals are attainable if you apply self discipline to achieve them, and I'm going to show you how. Always focus on the light at the end of the tunnel; look at the impact achieving your goals will have on your life once you have reached them. You can reach your goals if you think and believe you can!!

First, you need to know the difference between a LTG and a STG. A LTG is one you plan to reach within one to five years. Your STGs are going to be goals you can accomplish in less than one year that when accomplished, will lead you to accomplishing your LTGs. People make STGs by the hour, the day, the week, the month, a yearly quarter, and yearly.

We are focusing on weight loss goals right now. Once you make these goals and see how the process works, you can apply these same concepts and ideas to any other area of your life and accomplish anything you set out to do using these same methods you are going to use to lose and maintain your weight loss. So be thinking of other goals you have in your life that you want to apply these strategies to.

What is your LTG for loosing weight? How much total weight do you want to lose? What is a realistic time frame for this figuring a loss of one to two pounds per week? You've actually answered this question previously. We are just incorporating it into your plan now.

For example, there are fifty-two weeks in a year. One pound a week would be a weight loss of fifty-two pounds in one year; two pounds per week would be 104 pounds per year. So if you have one hundred pounds or more to lose, your LTG is going to be one year or greater. If you have less than one hundred pounds to lose, your LTG could be six or nine months. Your other LTG would be to maintain this weight loss for greater than one or five years. Once you reach the five year mark, you can extend your LTG for another five years.

Write your LTG something like this:

I will lose a total of one hundred pounds by (<u>date , one year from your start date</u>).

This goal is specific–you plan to lose one hundred pounds.

This goal is measurable — you will reach your goal one year from the date you put your plan into action.

Think of your LTG as "Your Mission."

Now for your STGs — they must be specific and measurable as well. Examples of what your STGs might read like are:

I will lose four to eight pounds per month or one to two pounds per week. I will accomplish this by:

> 1. Learning to read food labels and about the nutritional value of food and what my body

needs to become healthier and function properly.

2. I will implement lifestyle changes and set daily goals that will allow me to lose one to two pounds per week, maintain this weight loss upon reaching my LTG of one hundred pounds, and improve my health for life.

3. I will eat small, frequent, well-balanced meals, consisting mainly of vegetables, fruits, lean meat, complex carbohydrates, and low fat foods.

4. I will adjust the portions of the foods I eat to smaller, healthier sizes.

5. I will drink eight to nine glasses of water daily.

6. I will drink one 8 oz. glass of water thirty minutes before meals.

7. I will eat slowly and chew each bite thoroughly.

8. I will put my fork down and take a drink of water between each bite I eat to slow my eating.

9. I will only eat at the dining room table when eating at home.

10. I will not eat while driving or sitting in my car.

11. If I am eating out at a restaurant, I will order foods that are less energy dense and take half the food home with me to eat at a later time.

12. I will eat fruits or vegetables as snacks in place of snack foods from vending machines.

13. I will exercise three to five times per week. My exercise program will consist of walking, bike riding, stretching, and weight lifting for toning.

These are just examples of things you can do to reach your STGs. Later in the book, I have listed many, many strategies to use to help you lose weight. You need to read through these, pick a few that you think will work for you and use the ones you choose for your STGs.

After you have written down your LTGs and STGs, I want you to rewrite these in the form of a contract with yourself. Studies show that if you make a contract with yourself you are more committed to accomplishing your goals. This contract can be in the form of a "Personal Mission Statement." A Mission Statement is a simple statement of your purpose and goals that provides clarity and focus on what you want to accomplish. As I said earlier, you might think of your LTG as your mission. The Mission Statement is often followed by success criteria that states how you are going to accomplish your mission. These success criteria can be your STGs.

Remember as you make your STGs and LTGs, you must be willing to work hard and do what it takes to reach your goals. You will have to make changes to reach your goals. Be sure to ask yourself if your goals mean enough to you for you to be willing to work for them. Don't look at these changes as sacrifices, look at them as choices, positive choices. These choices and changes may be hard to make at first, but as they become part of your daily lifestyle, they will get easier and eventually you won't even think about returning to your old ways of eating. I like the way one person puts it. She says, "Thin feels better than fat. I wouldn't change that for anything."

Using the above example, your contract with yourself might read something like this:

I, Jane Smith deserve to be healthy. Beginning January 1, 2008, I will implement my plan to lose 100 pounds by January 1, 2009 through choices I make daily. My weight loss of 100 pounds will be accomplished in the following way:

I will lose four to eight pounds per month or one to two pounds per week by:

1. Learning to read food labels and learning about the nutritional value of food that my body needs to become healthier and function properly.
2. Implementing lifestyle changes and setting daily goals that will allow me to reduce my daily caloric intake by five hundred to one thousand calories and lose one to two pounds weekly and maintain this weight loss upon reaching my LTG of one hundred pounds, and improve my health for life.
3. Eating small, frequent, well-balanced meals consisting mainly of vegetables, fruits, lean meat, complex carbohydrates, and low fat foods.
4. Adjusting the portions of the foods I eat to smaller, healthier sizes.
5. Drinking a total of eight to nine, eight ounce glasses of water daily which includes drinking one eight ounce glass of water thirty minutes before meals.
6. Eating slowly and chewing each bite thoroughly.

7. Putting my fork down and taking a drink of water between each bite I eat in order to slow down my eating and allow my stomach to feel full.
8. Eating only at the dining room table when eating at home.
9. Not eating while driving or sitting in my car.
10. Choosing less energy dense foods when eating out at restaurants.
11. Asking for to-go boxes when I eat out at restaurants, taking half the food home with me to eat at a later time.
12. Eating fruits or vegetables as snacks in place of snack foods from vending machines.
13. Exercising three to five times per week consisting of walking, bike riding, stretching and weight lifting for toning.

Once you complete your LTGs and STGs, you want to set a start date. You will write this in your contract with yourself as in the above example.

Then what? What happens when you put your plan into action? Remember earlier I said that people who are successful achieving their goals look at them by the hour, the day, the week, the month, etc. I want you to review your progress weekly. This is the evaluation phase of your plan.

Let's use an example. Say you weigh yourself at the first of the week (Monday morning), and you weighed 152 pounds. Your goal is to lose one or two pounds per week, and you implemented the strategies we listed above. The next Monday morning, you weighed yourself, and you weigh 151 pounds. Great!! You lost a pound the previous week. So you reached your STG for the week. But don't stop here, review all the parts of your STGs. Perhaps you were going to walk thirty minutes three days last week and you only got to walk one of those days. Ask yourself, is this something I can realistically continue. If yes, recommit yourself to that STG. If not, change it to something you can do.

Go through each action you have listed. If one of them isn't working, change it or get rid of it. Remember, these are strategies you have to be able to implement and live with. If you are using strategies that aren't working or that you just can't do, they aren't going to work for the long term. Keep experimenting and trying different strategies until you come up with ones that become natural for you and you just do without thinking. Once you automatically do these things without thinking, you have changed your behavior permanently.

You may have days you totally "blow" your eating plan, we all do. But when this happens, that's ok. Just start over the next day, get back to your plan. If you are "blowing" your eating plan too often, start over and look at your whole plan. What do you need to change? Are you totally committed to reaching your goals? Ask yourself:

> W: "What do I want?"
> D: "What am I doing?"
> E: "Is it working?" Why or why not?
> P: "Do I need to change my plan?"

Reviewing your goals daily will help you achieve them. Set aside a few minutes every day to review your goals. Some people put aside some time in both the morning and the evening. In the morning, they make their STGs for the day. They may start off the day saying, "Just for today, I'm going to eat healthy and follow my plan of _____." In the evening, they will take a few minutes and review and evaluate what they did during the day and make changes as necessary. Reviewing your goals daily helps ingrain them into your subconscious mind and reminds your subconscious mind what you are working for. Your subconscious mind is a powerful force in helping you reach your goals. More about this later in the chapter on "Self Talk."

Hourly goals can help in stressful situations where you are tempted to stray from your weight management plan. For example, you are going to lunch with your coworkers, and you are going to your favorite restaurant, which serves your most favorite food in the whole world. You usually eat double portions of this food. You need to get through the next hour without "blowing" your plan. Here are some suggestions for STGs for the next hour.

1. Drink two glasses of water before going to the restaurant, and take one fiber capsule. Doing this will already partially fill up your stomach.
2. Don't order double portions.
3. Order a small salad as an appetizer with low fat dressing on the side, and eat this slowly as you wait for your meal.
4. Ask for a to-go box before you start eating and put half the food in the to-go box at the start of

the meal. Think about how good the second half of that is going to taste later.

5. Remember to chew each bite thoroughly and make yourself drink water between each bite.

6. Consciously slow down your eating. This will give your brain time to realize your stomach is full.

7. Savor each bite of your favorite food as you eat it. Think about how good it tastes and how much you are enjoying it as you slowly chew your food.

These are all strategies you already have listed in your STGs. Use them, but use all of them during that one hour that you know you are going to have a hard time getting through. If you do all these things and still eat more than you really should have, I bet you still have eaten less than you would have if you didn't use any of your strategies!

You have now made a behavioral contract with yourself to help you become self-disciplined to reach your goals. This behavioral contract is a promise to yourself. Read it daily. With this contract you have established external measures, your strategies, that you will use as inner resources to reach your goals. You have committed yourself to keeping your word to yourself as you would with any other contract you would make. Do the things you have listed in your contract for four to six weeks, and they will become habit. Once these things become habit, your commitment to achieving your goals will skyrocket.

Now we want to talk about rewards. You should always reward yourself when accomplish what you have set out to do. You have earned it. Rewards help reinforce the behavior you are trying to develop; the behavior you are trying to develop to take control of your life and succeed at what you want to accomplish.

To make your rewards use the Rewards Planner in the Appendix of the book or just take a piece of paper and draw a line down the middle. On the left side of the paper write "WHEN." On the right side of the paper write, "THEN." Your paper will look something like this:

WHEN   THEN

When I_____ then I can_____.

For example:
When I drink eight glasses of water a day, then I can drink one twelve oz. soda pop for the day.

When I lose two pounds, then I can go out to my favorite place to eat.

Beginning to get the idea? Link your rewards directly to your target behavior. You can also give yourself bonuses. For example:

When I lose ten pounds, I can buy a new pair of jeans.

Pair your rewards with your STGs and your bonuses with your LTGs. Bonuses are just a bigger reward once you reach several small goals.

A strategy some people use to help them reach their STGs and LTGs is with the use of tokens. Tokens can take the form of a penny, a paperclip, a poker chip, etc. A token is a symbol of what you are working for. For each glass of water you drink, put a token in a cup or small box. When you have eight tokens in the cup, then you can have your soda pop. When you lose your two pounds, put a token in the cup. When you have five of these tokens, you can go buy your pair of jeans. You may want to use different tokens to represent different things. The penny can represent the glasses of water. A paperclip can represent pounds. Your tokens themselves actually become rewards. Your token is your reward for drinking the one glass of water.

The next chapter is jammed full of strategies for you to use to succeed at your weight management plan. You can't use all of them. Read them, choose a few you think you can live with and implement them into your plan. Review and reevaluate your plan in a week. Keep what is working, and get rid of what is not working. Keep doing this weekly until everything you do is working for you, you are losing weight and accomplishing your STGs and your LTGs and maintaining your goal weight!

The great pleasure in life is doing what people say you cannot do.

Chapter nine

Living Your Plan

Now that you are starting to develop your weight loss and management plan, you need some proven strategies to help you get there. This chapter is full of more strategies than you will ever be able to use. You only need to use a few of them to make your plan successful. As you choose your strategies, remember that the changes you make are positive choices that will benefit you for the rest of your life. The choices you make will determine the life you lead.

As you implement your choices, there will be times your willpower will be tested and the going will be tough, but you have to be willing to make these changes to accomplish what you want. The self-discipline it takes to implement your changes will become easier, the more use practice it. Goals are attainable if you apply self-discipline to achieve them, and these goals can help you do things you never dreamed were possible. Remember, there are no unrealistic goals, only unrealistic time frames. You can accomplish anything with enough time.

One of the first strategies that I am going to suggest you use is to develop a support team. Research shows that people with support systems tend to be more successful in losing weight. Having support from others can help you stay motivated when the going gets tough. Support from others can also help affirm your belief in you and your goals.

You are going to get both positive and negative support from other people. It would be nice if all the support was positive, but it won't be. Many people will be happy with your efforts to lose weight, many will not be. The ones that don't support your efforts may attempt to interfere with your goals and your progress. The reasons for this negative support vary. Some may fear that their relationship with you will be changed or lost. Some will be jealous.

Wherever the negative support comes from and for whatever reason it is given, it can have an emotional and negative impact on you and your goals. Negative support can ruin your progress and your attempts to reach your goals. You are going to have to be tough to resist this influence.

How can you tell if someone is giving you negative support? Here are some examples. The person may tell you they "like you just the way you are," they "don't want you to change or lose weight." They may complain when you go for your daily walk or exercise activity. They may bring you cakes, cookies, candies, snacks, and all kinds of food you are trying to avoid. They may take you to your favorite restaurant and tell you that you can eat what you want, "just this one time." They may tell you that you can't do it or make remarks about your being "on another diet."

My response. You have to get tough and recognize what is happening. You have to be willing to put yourself first. Remember, when you look in the mirror every morning, you are looking at the person who is responsible for your weight and your health, your future, and your own security. Don't let anyone take that right away from you. Not anyone.

So what can you do to counteract this negative support? First, try to identify who these people are. My guess is you have already had some of this negative support from them in the past, so some of them will be easy to identify. Many of them will be your closest friends and your family. This is why you need a team that will give you positive support and that you can turn to when you feel overwhelmed by negative support.

So where do you find this support team? A good place to start is to find a friend or several friends who want to do the same thing you do. You might be able to find a community based weight reduction group through your work, church, or other club or organization. This enables you to work on your goals together, discuss new strategies for managing what you eat, and it provides you with someone to listen when the negative feedback hits you or when the going just gets tough.

Make a list of people who you think will support you and a list of those you think will not support you. Write down some of your strategies for dealing with negative feedback. If you have a plan in place, these situations will be easier to deal with. Develop your support team and stay close to them until you are strong enough to meet these challenges on your own.

There are also professional weight loss coaches available. There are actually several good weight loss programs on the market that provide a support team for you. This year, Consumer's Reports rated the top four weight loss programs on the market. They are:

> #1 – Volumetrics
> #2 – Weight Watchers
> #3 – Jenny Craig
> #4 – Slim for Life

The Volumetrics Weight Management program was developed by Barbara Rolls, Ph.D., a nutritionist. I don't know that this plan is commercially available, but her two books can be purchased at amazon.com. These are books I highly recommend. She does a wonderful job of teaching you how to eat more volume with less energy dense foods.

The other three programs do provide a support team for you. These work well for many people. Weight Watchers is one of my favorites. Over the years, I've seen people lose weight and keep it off with the Weight Watcher's program. I highly recommend this plan.

I offer weight loss coaching online, and you can find out more about my program at teresablancworld.com, or contact me at teresa@teresablancworld.com. Like my book, my coaching is based on Choice Theory and Reality Therapy. I help you develop a plan as outlined in this book and provide weekly discussion, guidance, and feedback by email. My coaching is probably more medically oriented than other programs since my background is as a Nurse Practitioner. I take your medical conditions into consideration while coaching you.

So start thinking about your support team and getting your team together. As you begin to develop your strategies, one of the first things you want to develop is a strategy for are the moments when your will power is tested. When you have one of these "will power challenging moments," remind yourself of your goals. Some people carry a list of their goals with them just for moments like this. Take the list of your goals out and read them. Remind yourself how important your goals are to you. Sit back, close your eyes, picture yourself reaching your goal weight and how you will look and feel and think about the things you will be able to do. Stall for time. The moment will pass. Make an hourly goal. Say, "just for the next hour I am not going to eat whatever the tempting food is." Write down what you are giving up and what you will get in return. Believe in and remind yourself of what you are trying to achieve. Look at and read your daily affirmations (see chapter on Self-Talk). Think about something else you accomplished in your life and how you felt when you accomplished it. Know this is how you will feel when you reach the weight loss goals you set for yourself.

Affirmation: "I am my own top priority."

Strategies for dealing with negative support

Be firm with these people. Never tell them you are "on a diet"; tell them you are eating healthier.

Thank them for their thoughts, but you will pass on the goodies this time.

Offer to let them have the cookies instead.

Just say, "No thank you."

Think about the day when you will be able to look at them and smile and say, "Look at me now. I did what I said I was going to do. I look good, and I feel good."

Strategies
Your Foundation

The foundation of a successful weight loss program starts with basic information. You need to estimate the number of calories you need per day. You need to know what portion sizes really are. You need to know what a balanced diet consist of.

A Balanced Diet

Your daily food intake should look something like this:

> Protein: 2 to 3 servings per day
> Dairy: 2 to 3 servings per day
> Fruit: 2 to 3 servings per day
> Vegetables: 4 to 6 servings per day

Whole grains: 5 to 6 servings per day
Fat: 1 to 3 servings of unsaturated fat per day

Estimating Ideal Body Weight:

For women: 100 pounds for the first 5 feet.
            Add 5 pounds for each additional inch.

For example, a female, 5'2" tall, the Ideal Body
Weight would be 110 pounds.

For men: 106 pounds for the first 5 feet.
            Add 6 pounds for each additional inch.

For example, a male, 5'10" tall, the Ideal Body
Weight would be 166 pounds.
(106 + 60 pounds = 166 pounds)

Estimating calories needed to maintain weight

For sedentary or obese individuals: 10 calories per
pound of desirable body weight.

For low physical activity or over 55 years old: 13 calories
per pound of desirable body weight.

For moderate physical activity: 15 calories per pound
of desirable body weight.

For strenuous physical activity 4 or 5 days per week: 18
calories per pound of desirable body weight.

For example, if you are a 56 y.o. person and your
desired body weight is 115 pounds, you would need

approximately 1,495 calories per day to maintain this weight. (115 pounds x 13 calories per pound = 1,495 calories).

The above formulas can be used as a guide for figuring an approximate number of calories needed per day. However, your caloric intake should never go below about 1,200 calories per day. Consuming fewer than 1,200 calories per day will throw your body into the survival mode where it thinks food is not available. Your body will slow your metabolism down to match what you are providing for it, and you will not lose weight. In fact, if you slow your metabolism down too much, you may even gain weight on 1,200 calories per day. That is why exercise and increasing activity is so important. Exercise and increasing your activity keep you burning calories and your metabolism functioning in a positive mode.

Recognizing When You are Hungry

You need to be able to recognize when you are hungry to be able to adjust what you are eating and lose weight. Not many of us know what real hunger is in this country. Food is available anytime, anyplace, 24 hours per day. Many people are overweight for the simple fact they "graze" all day long on some type of food and don't have distinct meal times.

So how do you know when you are really hungry? What does real hunger feel like? Your first step in learning what real hunger feels like is to allow enough time between eating periods to become hungry. Also, as you become more active and burn more calories, you will increase your ability to sense when you are hungry.

Try an experiment. Delay one of your meals until you feel actual hunger. You may have some physical discomfort initially. You may call this "stomach pain" or "abdominal pain." It will make you feel uncomfortable, especially if you haven't experienced this feeling before. Feeling uncomfortable is what is supposed to happen. This is your body's natural signal that it is time to eat. Once you know what hunger feels like, you want to use this feeling as a guide for eating, a guide to signal you that it is meal time. Write these feelings in your food diary. Record the times you feel actual hunger and note if there is a pattern to this. As you experience this feeling of hunger on a regular basis it should automatically become your signal for your meals.

Serving/Portion Sizes

Become familiar with what a serving or portion size looks like. Initially measure your food. After awhile you will unconsciously know what serving sizes look like.

A serving of meat, fish, or poultry should be about the size of the palm of your hand or the size of a deck of cards (about 3 ounces).

Fruit and vegetable portions should be about the size of your hand when it is cupped or about the size of a tennis or baseball (about ½ cup).

The tip of your thumb to the first joint = 1 tablespoon
The tip of your finger to the first joint = 1 teaspoon

Clenched fist = 1 cup
Cupped hand = ½ cup

One ounce of cheese = three dice (three 1 inch square cubes)

Six ounce (medium) apple = the size of a tennis or baseball

Six ounce (medium) baked potato = the size of a computer mouse

A slice of bread, one small roll, or a half a bagel or bun = one serving

Guidelines for putting food on your plate:

1. Use a plate smaller than you usually do — it will appear you have more food on your plate than you actually do. You will fool your subconscious mind. You will also be able to eat everything on your plate.
2. Mentally divide your plate into fourths: the main dish, meat or protein — ¼ of the plate; the bread or starch — ¼ of the plate; fruits and vegetables — ½ of the plate

Strategies to Reduce Fat in you Diet

Analyze your food diary and determine which foods you are currently eating that are high in fat. Determine if you are willing to eliminate these foods from your diet or decrease the amount of these foods in your diet.

Learn to read food labels to determine how much and what kind of fat a food contains. Work on eliminating the saturated and trans fats from your diet.

Purchase a fat gram counter. These are available where nutrition books are sold.

Don't keep high fat foods at home, especially snack foods.

Cook with olive or canola oil.

Choose lean cuts of meat and poultry; trim off excess fat before cooking.

Avoid fried foods.

Eat more chicken, turkey, and fish, and less red meat.

Avoid processed lunch meats such as bologna, salami, hotdogs, etc.

Use low-fat milk and cheeses.

Eat more fruits and vegetables.

Use vinegar and oil type salad dressings.

Eat fruit, sorbet, ice milk, berries, and angel food cake for desserts.

Add high fiber and complex carbohydrate foods to your diet.

If you eat a meal with a large amount of fat, add fiber foods to that meal. Fat and cholesterol bind to fiber and get passed out of the body in the stool instead of being absorbed by the body.

Strategies for meal times and snacks

Make meals a special activity, a time to sit down and focus on eating and not something to be rushed through.

> Results of rushing through meals: You eat so fast there isn't time for your mind to tell your stomach when you are full and you overeat.

> You don't have time to enjoy what you are eating and may not even think about what you are eating. This is called "mindless eating."

> You don't have time to enjoy the company of the person you are with.

Organize your meals into three meals and two snacks

Meals and snacks should be something to look forward to. Eating should be "quality time" for you and the person you are with.

Make mealtime and snack time pleasant—play music, burn candles, have friends join you.

Eat slowly. Savor your food. Enjoy each bite.

(Eating slowly should be one of your strategies to decrease your food intake. It takes 10 to 15 minutes for the signal to get from your stomach to your brain that you have had enough to eat. Eating slowly provides this time.)

Chew your food thoroughly. Chew each bite of food 10 to 20 times before swallowing.

Put your fork down between each bite and swallow your food before picking your fork back up.

To make your stomach feel fuller, take a swallow of water between each bite. This slows your eating down. It also provides volume, which makes your stomach think it is full.

Drink one or two glasses of water prior to your meal to fool your stomach into thinking it is full.

Take a fiber pill with your two glasses of water prior to your meals. This provides bulk, fiber, and no calories as well as filling your stomach up.

(CAUTION! Make sure you drink eight to sixteen ounces of water with fiber pills. The fiber swells in your stomach. If you do not drink enough water with each pill, there is a chance the fiber will solidify in your stomach or intestines, causing constipation or a bowel obstruction. Also, if you are not used to having a significant amount of fiber in your diet, you may initially have loose stools or diarrhea after taking these fiber pills. Their medical classification is that of a bulk laxative. If you do develop loose stools or diarrhea, just cut down on the number of fiber pills you are using per day. As your body gets used to the fiber in your new diet, the loose stools will be corrected, and you will just have normal, soft, formed bowel movements.)

Second helpings: Want second helpings? Wait 10 or 15 minutes before actually doing so. If you are still hungry and need something else to eat, take a second helping of the fruits or vegetables rather than the higher calorie foods or dessert.

Breakfast

Breakfast really is the most important meal of the day. Research shows that people who eat breakfast tend to lose weight faster and keep it off longer than those who skip breakfast; however, only 49% of people in the United States eat breakfast every day.

People who skip breakfast typically eat 200 to 300 more calories per day than those who eat breakfast. People who skip breakfast tend to have a lower metabolic rate than people who eat breakfast. Why? Eating breakfast helps you keep your metabolism at a higher level, which means you will burn more calories throughout the day. After sleeping, your body has been fasting for several hours. You need glucose for energy for your body and brain to start functioning after this fasting period. Breakfast provides this energy.

Breakfast doesn't have to be eaten as soon as you get out of bed. You can wait till you feel like eating and are hungry. Let your body tell you when you are hungry and ready to eat.

It is good to put fiber in your diet at breakfast. Foods high in fiber help you feel full longer and are usually low in calories. If you feel full longer, you will eat fewer snacks and eat less at your next meal. There are many good breakfast foods on the market that are high in fiber. Examples of high fiber cereals are oatmeal, Fiber One, Raisin Brand, and Wheat Chex.

Try to stay away from high fat foods at breakfast time. These include foods like bacon and sausage. Try substituting low-fat turkey bacon, Canadian bacon, or ham for these.

Drink coffee black. Black coffee has no calories. When you put sugar and cream in coffee, you can potentially add as much as 400 or 500 calories. If you drink a lot of coffee, consider cutting down on the amount you consume as there are health risks associated with high caffeine intake, including high blood pressure and coronary artery disease.

Eat fruit instead of drinking juice at breakfast. The very act of chewing helps your body recognize when it is full. You don't get this recognition when you drink liquids. Chewing the fruit takes longer than drinking a glass of juice, giving your body that time it needs to send the signal of feeling full from your stomach to your brain. There is also the risk of getting more calories from juice than from fresh fruit. Many processed juices (canned, bottled, etc.) have sugar added to them. Also fresh fruits have more fiber than juice does.

Lunch

The first rule for eating lunch is to eat breakfast. If you don't eat breakfast, you are likely to be starving by lunch time and to eat many more calories than you need.

The second rule for lunch is not to wait until you are starving to eat. If you are always starving by lunch time, then add a midmorning healthy snack to your eating routine. Remember, we said your daily eating patterns should include three meals and two snacks. The midmorning snack can be one of these.

Many people eat out at lunch due to working away from home. Bring lunch from home if you can. Your lunch will probably be healthier and contain fewer calories, and you will save money in the process. If you can't bring your lunch, then you will want to develop some strategies to help you limit the number of calories consumed at lunch.

Again, don't arrive at a restaurant starved. If you do, and they serve bread or chips before the meal, you will usually end up eating too much of this food. Consider asking that bread or chips not be served; however, if you are with other people, this may not be an option. Ask for fresh fruit as an appetizer. Know your meal plan. Think about what you are going to do ahead of time. Try to eat lunch within an hour of the same time each day. It is easier to control your appetite if you eat at approximately the same time each day. This same strategy can be used for other meals as well.

If you haven't eaten at a restaurant before, consider contacting them ahead of time and ask if they will be able to meet your dietary requirements. For example, say you want to order something broiled instead of fried. Many restaurants now have a web site where you can actually look at the menu in advance to see what types of foods are served. Some may have nutritional information online also. Study the menu carefully for light or lighter choices.

Lunch time is a good time to eat your largest meal of the day. This gives you time in the afternoon to work off some of those calories eaten at lunch. Then eat a smaller meal in the evening.

Ask the restaurant for a listing of the calorie counts for the foods they serve. This is especially important if you eat at the same restaurant frequently. Many restaurants have these now with people trying to eat healthier. Some cafeterias have started putting up signs with the nutritional values of the foods that are being served. If you don't see this nutritional information though, ask for it. Knowing the nutritional information of the foods served will help you in choosing the lower calorie items. Try eating similar foods each day, but not the same. Eating similar foods will help prevent you from eating extra calories when you are in a hurry, but eating the same foods would be very boring and make it harder to stick to your plan.

Eat large salads at lunch or anytime you are eating out (green salad, not pasta or bean salad). Use oil and vinegar type dressings if possible as these are usually lower in calories. Otherwise, use low calorie salad dressings. Be careful about low fat salad dressings as many of them contain sugar in place of the fat and almost as many calories as the regular dressings. Ask for salad dressing on the side. Use it sparingly, whichever type you use. Salsa is a good low-fat substitute for salad dressing.

When eating out at restaurants, be aware that one restaurant portion will often equal two or three regular portions. When you order, go ahead and ask for a to-go box, and before you even start to eat, put half the order in the box to take with you. You will cut the calories in half right from the start. You will also save some money as this can be used for another meal at a later time. If you think you will be tempted to eat all your order, you can ask the server to place half the order in the box before bringing the food to the table and bring the box to you at the end of the meal when you are ready to leave.

Consider splitting your meal with the person you are with. Some restaurants frown on this and will be reluctant to provide you with an additional place setting of silverware, but it is worth a try.

If the restaurant will allow it, order a child's portion. Then you can eat the entire order and not have to worry about the to-go box.

Once you get used to eating these smaller portions, it will become habit. You will ask for the to-go box out of habit. Also, you will find you don't even want all the food that is brought to you when you become used to the smaller portions. You will feel full when you have consumed the smaller amount.

When reading the menu at a restaurant, look at it carefully. The description of the food often tells how it is prepared. If in doubt as to how the food is prepared, ask the server. Ask if the food can be prepared differently so as to contain fewer calories. Many restaurants will do this. Don't hesitate to ask—you are the paying customer. All they can do is say no.

If possible, order a la cart. This way you only order what you want and don't end up with a lot of extra things on your plate that will be a temptation to eat. The disadvantage here is that sometimes this will cost more.

If you drink coffee, ask for skim or low fat milk instead of cream.

Choose beverages carefully—stay away from drinks with sugar (soft drinks, sweetened tea, fruit drinks).

Ordering steak or another piece of meat, ask that all visible fat be trimmed from the meat prior to cooking it.

Have skin removed from chicken prior to cooking. Order baked chicken breast when possible.

Entrée with sauce: ask if the sauce can be served on the side.

Select fresh fruit as an appetizer or dessert.

Vegetables—ask if they can be steamed rather than cooked in oil or butter.

Don't super size your meals.

<u>Menu tips</u>

Try these for appetizers:
> Fresh vegetables
> Garden salads
> Broth soups
> Unbuttered wheat bread
> Rye crackers or crisps

These will be low fat:
> Steamed
> Garden fresh
> Roasted
> Broiled
> Poached
> Tomato juice
> In its own juice

These will be high in calories or fat:
> Fried
> Crispy
> Hash

Gravy
Creamed
Buttery
Butter sauce
Au Gratin
Escalloped
Hollandale
Parmesan

Try these for dessert:
Fresh fruits
Angel food or sponge cake
Sherbet
Ice milk

Try these for beverages:
Water
Unsweetened tea or coffee
Diet soda pop
Tomato or V-8 juice

Dinner

Make dinner a smaller meal than your noon meal if possible. If you eat a large lunch, don't eat a large dinner meal.

Eat your evening meal at least two to three hours before bedtime. You want to be able to burn some of these calories before you go to sleep.

Strategies to avoid eating too fast:

The purpose of eating slowly is to give your stomach time to recognize there is food in it and convey this message to your brain. This process takes 10 to 15 minutes. If you eat too quickly, you will have stuffed your stomach before it has had any time to communicate with your brain.

After your food is placed in front of you, wait five minutes before you start eating.

Chew your food completely before swallowing it (10 to 20 chews per bite).

Put your eating utensil down between bites.

Cutting meat? Cut one bite at a time, and eat this bite before cutting another bite.

Take a drink of water between bites.

Swallow each bite completely before picking up more food to eat.

Only put small amounts of food on your eating utensil.

Use smaller utensils such as a cocktail fork to avoid shoveling food into your mouth. Use a teaspoon instead of a soup spoon for the same reason.

Make your meals last longer; stretch them out to thirty minutes to allow time to savor your food and reduce your hunger.

Wait several minutes between courses in your meal.

When you have finished what is on your plate, wait 10 to 15 minutes before taking any second helpings (then follow the previous strategies for eating second helpings).

Strategies to avoid eating oversized portions:

Measure your food.

Learn portion sizes as noted earlier in the chapter.

Use smaller plates for your meals.

Purchase single-serving foods.

Don't super size your meals.

Strategies to avoid eating leftovers:

Put all extra food away as you prepare your meal.

Don't serve your food at the table. By serving your food before you get to the table the extra food isn't sitting there to tempt you.

Get up and leave the table when you are finished eating your first helping.

Let someone else clean up the leftovers and put them away.

Get into the habit of leaving some food on your plate.

Prepare or buy food in smaller quantities, so you don't have leftovers.

Immediately freeze any leftovers for future use, so they are not in the refrigerator to tempt you.

Strategies to avoid grazing:

Grazing is constant nibbling or munching on food all day long without really thinking about what you are eating – sometimes referred to as "mindless eating."

Get rid of snack food in your home or if unable to do this put it out of site.

Select one area of your home to eat in and avoid eating in other locations. Anytime you eat in your home, eat in this location.

Never eat while reading or watching television (mindless eating).

Never eat in your car.

Do not stand in front of the refrigerator or cabinet and eat.

Do not eat on the run. Don't eat if you don't have time to sit down and think about what you are eating and enjoy it.

Don't sample food that you are cooking. Chewing sugar-free gum helps here.

If you do sample food, don't forget to count the calories and add this to your food diary.

Minimize the time you spend in the kitchen.

Strategies to avoid bedtime snacking:

Make a rule that you will not eat within two hours of bedtime.

Brush your teeth after dinner. This signals your body that you are through eating for the day.

Pick a certain time of day that you will not eat after.

Don't eat in front of the television, while reading or while sitting in bed.

Strategies to avoid overeating at social events:

Eat fruit or vegetables before the event.

Drink one or two glasses of water before the event.

Take a fiber pill with the two glasses of water before the event.

Concentrate on the people at the event and not the food.

Stay away from the food table.

Keep moving and mingling instead of eating. Mingle, mingle, mingle.

Keep talking—you won't eat if you are talking.

Strategies to help control cravings:

Try to determine if there is a trigger associated with your cravings. A trigger is something that happens, things you see or do that make you want a certain food. For example, for some people, commercial time on the television is trigger for them to get something to eat, especially if the commercial is advertising food. Learn what your triggers are and avoid them if possible.

Incorporate foods you crave into your diet on a regular basis.

When a craving is triggered, eat only a small portion of it. For example, if you are craving chocolate, eat a chocolate kiss or miniature chocolate bar instead of a large one. Each milk chocolate kiss has 25 calories, and the small chocolate bars average about 45 calories. Don't forget to write this in your food diary.

Select the healthiest version of the food you crave. For example, craving ice cream, choose ice milk, sherbet, or the flavored ice instead.

Don't try substituting another food for the food you crave. You will probably just end up eating both.

Try substituting other pleasurable activities for the craved food.

Keep your hands busy. If you like to knit or crochet, do this while watching television to keep your hands busy and mind off eating.

Eat your meal on a regular schedule at about the same time each day. Don't forget your two healthy snacks that should be planned into your eating schedule.

Practice substitution when possible. For example, one tablespoon of mayo has about 90 calories. One tablespoon of mustard has no calories.

Cook chicken with the skin off. Chicken is higher in fat if it is cooked with the skin on.

Strategies to help you feel full or satisfied:

Drink 1 or 2 glasses of water prior to your meal.

Take 1 or 2 fiber pills with your 2 glasses of water.

Take a swallow of water between each bite.

Add water to food whenever possible to increase the volume of what you are eating.

Add vegetables to your recipes to increase the volume of low energy dense, low calories food in the recipe.

Add vegetables and fruits to the menu to increase the volume of low energy dense, low calorie foods in your meal.

Eat slowly to allow time for your brain to get the signal that there is food in your stomach.

Increase the amount of fiber foods in your recipes and your meals.

Strategies to avoid emotional eating:

Organize your eating into 3 meals and 2 snacks daily.

Make eating a conscious activity.

Learn what real hunger feels like (described above).

Identify the reasons and occasions that you eat out of emotion. Write your thoughts in your food diary.

If you are depressed, consider seeking professional counseling.

Use emotional eating to learn what needs to change in your life.

Learn to recognize reasons for emotional eating: boredom, stress, loneliness, emotional turmoil, or depression, and set goals to change these things in your life, using the same format and plan you are using to lose weight. Make a goal and determine the steps you need to take to achieve your goal.

Conclusion:

All of the above strategies will not work for everyone, but you should be able to pick out several that will work for you and will make a tremendous difference in the amount of food you eat and the number of calories you consume. The strategies you choose should be manageable, moderate, and promote a feeling of success in your weight loss and management plan. It only takes a few of these strategies incorporated into your daily eating habits to make your weight loss plan a success.

Plateaus

A plateau is when you stop losing weight for a period of time. You may even gain a few pounds. This is your body's way of maintaining its fat storage.

You have to have a certain amount of body fat to live. Body fat is used to protect internal organs, insulate you from the cold, and as a reserve source of energy. Your body has built-in mechanisms to prevent you from losing essential fat too quickly.

When you reach a plateau, it is time to change something about your weight loss program. You may need to reanalyze your food diary and make adjustments in your food consumption. You may need to increase your exercise or change to a different type of exercise for awhile. You may need to change some of your strategies.

You probably will not reach a plateau during the first 6 to 8 weeks. Your body will be adjusting to your new eating patterns and exercise pattern during this time. If you have been consistently loosing weight and your weight loss stops for at least 3 weeks, you may have hit a real plateau. Be patient. Don't quit. Analyze where you are at in relation to where you are going. Make some changes and see if this helps. The plateau will eventually pass, and you will start losing weight again.

Don't become discouraged. Continue reviewing your goals daily, using your strategies and keep yourself motivated with your support team and your daily self-talk.

Setbacks

A setback is something that occurs to temporarily stop or interrupt your progress toward your goal. Setbacks happen to everyone no matter how good your plan is for reaching your goals. The best way to look at these setbacks is to think of them as challenges and a natural part of your progress. Challenges add meaning to your life and represent opportunities for you to grow. When you overcome your setbacks and reach your goals, you will have a wonderful sense of accomplishment.

Be prepared for setbacks. They may come in the form of a plateau that takes several weeks to get through, muscular soreness and body aches that temporarily prevent you from exercising, family and work commitments, and many other things that keep your plan from working as smoothly as you would like. These things can discourage you and make you want to give up and quit. Don't let them!

Keep a positive attitude and never, never give up or quit! Maintaining a positive attitude and maintaining the belief that you can do whatever it takes to reach your goals needs to become the core of your plan and what your objectives revolve around. Review your goals daily, use self-talk, visualize yourself reaching your goals and seek support from your support team when setbacks occur.

Try the following:
Describe a "can't."
Now describe a "can."
There isn't such a thing as a "can't."

Make yourself an "I can."
Take a vegetable can with the label removed. Look through magazines and cut out all the pictures of glasses and eyes you can find. Glue these on your can, completely covering the outside of the can. Let dry.
You now have an "I can."
Sit this where you can see it and be motivated by it.

Chapter Ten

Physical Activity

A physical activity and exercise program is often the downfall of someone trying to lose weight. Many people do not enjoy exercise or have just not found an exercise they enjoy. Many people say they don't have time to exercise. And, unfortunately, if you are overweight or obese, you may not have the energy or stamina to exercise. This will make exercise more difficult for you.

Like it or not, physical activity is the way to kick your metabolism into high gear and lose weight faster. Physical activity also allows you to eat more food because you are burning more calories during the day.

Physical activity tones your muscles, makes them stronger, makes you look better, improves the function of many of your internal organs (especially the heart), helps you become more healthy in general, and helps prevent many chronic diseases.

One way to lose weight is to not change anything you eat, just find a way to burn an additional 500 calories per day. It takes 3,500 calories to make a pound, so by burning an additional 500 calories per day you burn an extra 3,500 calories per week and lose 1 pound per week. If you cut 500 calories per day out of your diet and burn an additional 500 calories per day through physical activity, you will lose 2 pounds per week.

Aerobic exercise is the type of exercise that helps you most in burning additional calories. It is also the type of exercise that increases your cardiovascular fitness and helps increase your metabolism so you burn more calories. You want to make aerobic exercise the foundation of your fitness routine.

Another kind of exercise is strength training. Strength training focuses on certain muscles groups, improving the function of these muscles. Strength training is important, but to burn the calories and improve cardiovascular health you still want to focus on the aerobic exercise.

When you perform an aerobic exercise, you are increasing your body's need for oxygen. This increased need for oxygen makes your heart beat faster and your respiratory rate faster. As this happens your body produces and stores aerobic enzymes that help you to burn fat and calories. Examples of aerobic exercises are walking, jogging, running, swimming, and bicycle riding.

When you are inactive and don't exercise, your body loses this ability to burn extra oxygen and calories. People usually say they are "out of shape" when this occurs. It takes a while to get "back in shape" when you start an exercise program.

Some type of physical activity needs to be added to your plan for weight loss and weight management. My favorite and the one I encourage people to use is just plain walking. Walking can be done anywhere, indoors or outdoors, and can be done every day. Walking is free. It doesn't cost anything to walk. There is minimal risk for injury. Walking can be done at your own speed and pace. Walking is something almost everyone can do. Walking is fun, easy, and best of all, it works!

Although it is easy, if you aren't used to walking, it and natural, just like the changes you are making in your eating habits aren't natural and comfortable at the beginning. Plan on about 6 to 8 weeks of walking will take awhile for walking to feel comfortable three times a week before it feels natural to you. In six months, walking will be a habit, and you won't want to give it up.

Before you begin walking be sure you are wearing comfortable clothes and good walking shoes. Good walking shoes are very important for giving your feet and your body proper support. Your shoes should have good arch and heel support, and there should be plenty of room for your toes. When you are overweight, you are already putting extra stress on your feet, so do everything you can to help your feet in your new endeavor. Before you begin a walking or other exercise program, make sure you have had your physical exam by your health care provider as discussed earlier in the book.

When you start your walking program, plan to begin by walking three times a week for about 20 minutes each session. Alternate your walking days. Walk every other day. National guidelines encourage people to exercise most days of the week. You will build up to this as you get use to walking.

Drink plenty of water before, during and after your walk to replace the fluids lost as you exercise. There are many nice carriers for water bottles on the market to use while exercising. These can be found at sports, hiking, and bicycle shops.

Walk at a pace that allows you to talk and breath at the same time. You don't want to get out of breath while walking. If you do, this means you need to slow down. I'll show you how to use your heart rate as a guide to exercise shortly.

You have probably heard you need to warm up before you exercise. This is as true with walking as with any other exercise. You may want to do some stretching exercises. This will help prevent pulled muscles and sprained ankles while walking. Also, begin your walk with a five minute, slow, warm-up walk, then walk briskly, and end your walk with another five minute, slow, cool-down walk. Some people end their walk with additional stretching exercises.

Properly warming up with stretching exercises and a five minute warm-up walk helps prevent injury to cold and stiff muscles. It also helps produce a slight rise in body temperature, which helps the muscles meet the metabolic demands of walking.

The cool-down walk has similar functions. During the five minute cool-down walk, your heart rate slows back to normal levels. This helps with removal of lactic acid from the muscles which helps reduce muscle soreness and stiffness later. Cool-down walking should be done until your breathing and pulse rate return to normal.

Another trick to helping prevent muscular soreness, if you are less than 50 years old and do not have any kidney disease or insufficiency, is to take a couple of Ibuprofen pain relievers before you exercise. Ibuprofen is an anti-inflammatory pain reliever. Taking Ibuprofen prior to exercising helps prevent inflammation from occurring as you exercise.

People older than 50 or those who have renal insuffiency or any type of kidney disease should use extreme caution when taking Ibuprophen and other nonsteroidal anti-inflammatory pain medications as these medications can have side effects which can make renal insufficiency or kidney disease worse.

If you are walking in the summer, consider walking in the early morning or evening. Temperatures are cooler then. If the temperature is greater than 90 or the humidity greater than 80%, then walk indoors at the gym or at a mall. The reverse is true in the winter. If it is below freezing, walk indoors. Also, during the winter you want to wear a hat, scarves, gloves and light layers of clothing that you can remove as your body warms up.

When walking on a highway, always walk against the traffic, meaning walk facing the oncoming traffic. If you are walking with other people, walk single file when there is traffic to contend with.

Try to walk during the daylight hours, but if you must walk at night, walk in a well-lighted area and wear reflective clothing and carry a flashlight. Flash lights are available now that you can wear on your head, and they point in the exact direction you are walking.

Don't feel like you have to walk fast or win a race. You want to walk naturally and have fun doing it. If your choice of exercise isn't fun, you won't like doing it and will not do it for very long.

When you walk, walk with your head erect. Look about 12 feet in front of you. Walk using good posture but walk relaxed. Lean forward slightly when you walk up or down hills for better balance. Swing your arms back and forth as you walk, but do this naturally. Swinging your arms back and forth gives more power and distance to your stride, helps you keep your balance, and helps you burn more calories.

There is a type of walking called "Fitness Walking." This is the same as normal walking, except you bring your forearms up to a 90 degree angle and lock in at the elbows and the hands in a loosely-clenched fist with thumbs on top. In Fitness Walking, your arms function for balance and as a guide which counter balances your forward motion and sets the timing of your steps. When your walking speeds up, you reach a steady pace and move into a striding gait.

If you haven't exercised in a long time, don't start your walking program by trying to walk a long distance. Start out with a 10 or 15 minute walk and gradually increase your walking time until you can walk as long as you like without tiring. This may take several months, and that is ok. Remember you are doing this for you and doing it at your own pace. You start where you are, not where someone else thinks you should be.

Many people are using pedometers now when they walk. A pedometer is a little device that you wear on your belt that records how many steps you walk per day. I know people who make a goal of walking so many steps per day, and when they can reach their goal daily, they continue to increase the number of steps. If you decide to use one of these, wear it for a few days to see how many steps you are usually walking, and then make your goal above what you normally walk.

The number of calories you burn while you walk depends on your weight and your speed. The chart below can be used as a guide to how many calories you are burning.

Speed/ pounds	100 lbs.	120 lbs.	140 lbs.	160 lbs.	180 lbs.	200 lbs.	220 lbs.	250 lbs.	275 lbs.	300 lbs.
2.0 mph	57	68	80	91	102	114	125	142	156	170
2.5 mph	55	65	76	87	98	109	120	136	150	164
3.0 mph	53	64	74	85	95	106	117	133	146	159
3.5 mph	52	62	73	83	94	104	114	130	143	156
4.0 mph	57	68	80	91	102	114	125	142	156	170
4.5 mph	64	76	89	102	115	127	140	159	175	191
5.0 mph	73	87	102	116	131	145	160	182	200	218

There is a guide you can use to determine a safe walking speed for yourself. It is referred to as "The Zone" and is used as a guide for judging the intensity of aerobic exercise. The zone is the intensity of exercise that safely produces the results you want. If you exercise below the ideal zone, you may not get the results you want from your exercise program. If you work above the zone, you may get tired too quickly and not get the maximum benefit from your exercise or you may injure yourself.

This technique can be used by calculating your "target heart rate." The target heart rate is the recommended range of heart rates (in beats per minute) that you should achieve during your exercise in order to safely train your cardiovascular system.

To determine your target heart rate:

> **Subtract your age from 220.** This is your maximum heart rate. You do not want your heart rate to go above this for any extended period of time.

> **Multiply this rate by .80 (80%)**. This is your target heart rate.

> **To estimate your target heart range,** add 5 (beats) to your target heart rate and subtract 5 (beats) from your target heart rate.

Example:
>Estimated maximum heart rate:
>>220 - 40 = 180 beats per minute

Target heart rate:
>180 x .80 =144 beats per minute

Target range:
>(144 - 5 = 139) and (144 + 5 = 149)
>139 to 149 beats per minute is the target range.

You want to stay in this target range when you are walking or exercising. To find out if you are in this range, stop every so often and check your carotid pulse. You will feel this in your neck either to the right or left of your Adam's apple. (Do not feel both right and left carotid arteries at the same time. This will occlude both of them, cut off the blood supply to your head, and you will pass out). Check the carotid pulse for six seconds, and multiple this by 10 to get your heart rate per minute. If your heart rate is slower than your target heart rate range, speed up the rate you are walking at. If your heart rate is above your target range, then slow your walking down.

There are many aerobic exercises out there besides walking that you can choose from. Find one you like or think you might like and try it. Don't limit yourself to one. Do any form of exercise you enjoy, combine them for variety and overall fitness. Consider adding strength training to your exercise program to help tone and define your muscles.

After you choose your activity program, make goals as you did for your eating program and add these to make your total program. Review your exercise goals weekly just as you review your eating plan weekly and make adjustments as necessary.

If you lose your dreams, you die inside.
Don't let anyone steal your dreams.

Chapter Eleven

Self-Talk: Affirmations

What is an affirmation? An affirmation is a positive, powerful belief, thought or statement that a person uses to allow the manifestation of that person's destiny. Affirmations are thoughts to support your goals and keep you motivated. An affirmation is a thought you choose to think because you like the results it will produce for you.

I'm going to teach you to use affirmations to help you lose weight and improve your health, but affirmations can be used in any area of your life and for reaching any goal. Remember I said earlier that you can use this same plan you are using to lose weight to achieve any other goal you have in life. You can use affirmations to help you lose weight and to reach any kind of goal you choose and to help eliminate negativity.

Affirmations are related to a psychological concept and technique called Biofeedback. Biofeedback was developed by Neal Miller, a psychologist and neuroscientist at Yale University during the middle of the 20th century. He experimented with rats and found that it was possible to train them to control their bodily functions such as heart rate, blood pressure and body temperature. Since that time much research has been done in understanding the mechanism of self-regulation of the body. Biofeedback is used today in pain management, stress reduction and many other areas. Comparing affirmations to biofeedback can help you understand how they work.

So how do you make and use affirmations? First, decide what area of your life you want to work on. In this case, the area you want to work on is losing weight, maintaining that weight loss, and becoming healthier in the process. Second, make positive statements to support the goal you want to work on. For example, some affirmations you might want to use for your weight loss program are:

> "I deserve to be healthy — I am healthy."
> "I have the power to control my health and my weight."
> "I have abundant energy, vitality, and well-being."
> "I control my own body."
> "I control my own destiny."
> "I am able to obtain and maintain my ideal weight."
> "I have sufficient energy for all my daily activities."
> "I love and care for my body, and it cares for and takes care of me."

Skeptical? Before you say, "That won't work" try an experiment. Every day, spend a few minutes telling yourself you are going to contract some dreaded disease or that you are going to be in an automobile accident. Don't want to do it? Why not? You don't want to do it because you have some belief that this will really happen and these things are things you don't want to happen — they are negative things. These are negative affirmations, but they are affirmations. Negative affirmations work as well as positive affirmations.

If you did the experiment above, probably one or two things would happen. Over a few days' time you would probably find yourself becoming very negative, in a bad mood, worrying. You would be giving yourself negative self talk, and it would start to affect you and what was happening in your life. If you did this long enough, it would affect your health. You might start having a few more aches and pains, maybe headaches and worst of all, you might develop some unwanted disease. Research studies have shown that a positive attitude makes a big difference in the outcome of people with cancer and other chronic diseases. With a positive attitude these people often live longer than was anticipated with fewer complications of the disease process, and many are even cured of their disease. A positive attitude does make a difference.

Self talk and affirmations are not new. Earl Nightingale, a motivational speaker from the 1950s and 1960s, said in his talk, "The Strangest Secret," "You become what you think about." Examples of this are all around us. For example, the person who may not have been very popular in high school but had the desire and determination to do something in life shows up at a class reunion ten or twenty years down the road and is the only millionaire from the group. From the same class, the person voted most likely to succeed might be on unemployment and can't keep a job. This person's thoughts may have been centered more around having a good time and being popular.

You become what you think about. That is why affirmations work. If you change your thoughts, you can change the direction of your life. All your thoughts affirm something. Use this affirmation, "The way I think can help me achieve all my goals."

In making affirmations, after you decide what area of your life you want to work on, decide what you want your affirmations to be. Your affirmations should be in the present or past tense. Don't use future tense. You are telling your subconscious the event has already happened. Use the most positive terms you know or can think of. NEVER use negative terms.

Write your affirmations down. You want to remember them exactly word-for-word. They should be short and specific. Personalize them by using "I" or use your name. Believe in them. Believe they are happening. The more you believe, the more powerful they become. Use repetition. Repetition drives them into your subconscious.

Review and say or write your affirmations daily. Call them "Daily Affirmations." This helps set a pattern for you, so you will use them daily. Review them at the same time you review the goals you have made. Reviewing them at this time helps affirm your goals. As you say your Daily Affirmations, practice seeing yourself in a new, more positive way.

Affirmations are powerful because they are simple and make a difference. They are like seeds that you plant in the soil in the garden of your mind. Plant your affirmations in your mind, nourish them daily, and watch them grow and develop.

Now make some affirmations of your own. Use the ones above to help get you started. Try your affirmations for a month, along with your new weight loss plan. Write them down. Read your affirmations and your goals daily. Then trust them, they will work for you.

As with your weight loss plan, your affirmations must be reviewed and reevaluated from time to time. You may reach a plateau. As you change, you may reach a point where you feel like you are getting stuck, much like a plateau you might reach loosing weight. Change them to make them more workable as necessary but don't give up on them.

Remember what Earl Nightingale said, "You become what you think about."

We are what we repeatedly do. Excellence, then, is not an act, but a habit.
-Aristotle

Chapter Twelve

Success and Not So Successful Stories

As a Nurse Practitioner I have had many, many patients seeking information on how to lose weight and keep it off. I have given lots and lots of advise – sound advise. However, I found a very large number of my patients weren't really looking for the sound advise, but were looking for the short cut to weight loss. Seems like everyone wants that magic weight loss pill.

Many years ago there were weight loss drugs on the market called amphetamines, also known as "speed." These were effective for many people, but there were also some very deadly side effects associated with them. Also, many people used them for other than their intended purpose, such as staying up for days without going to sleep. These were eventually taken off the market.

When I first got out of graduate school there were several new weight loss medications on the market. These promised to be very effective medications and people were successfully losing weight with them. Then it was discovered that many people who used them were developing a deadly disease called Pulmonary

Hypertensive. Again, the medications were removed from the market.

I continued to be asked about weight loss and I continued to give advise. I had developed a little meal plan and daily walking plan that I gave to patients when they asked about weight loss, hoping that they would put this plan into action. One day I was seeing a patient at the clinic and this patient had a friend with her. Her friend said to me, "You don't remember me, do you?" Obviously I did not. The girl, I'll call her Jane, was in her mid 20's, slim and very healthy looking. Jane went on to tell me that about a year prior to that she had been in to see me and had asked me about losing weight. I had given her my little plan I had developed. Jane took the information I gave her and started using the information. She said she followed the guidelines for eating, which were basically cut down on portion sizes and fat in the diet and exercise regularly, which was to walk daily. In the year after I gave her the plan Jane lost almost 100 pounds. At the time I was talking with her she had 20 more pounds to lose to reach her goal. She had come to the clinic with her friend to thank me for giving her that information. My first success story and the one that has left the biggest impression in my mind. I was excited!!! I had actually made a difference in this person's life. A big difference!! Her whole life changed for the better because of that weight loss. It was then that I decided I wanted to help other people achieve the same success this one patient had had.

Following are a few more stories of people that have and have not lost weight by making goals and a plan and sticking to it. My purpose in sharing the stories with you is to help you know that other people, just like you, have accomplished the same things you want to. It can be done. You can do it if you think you can and are willing to put forth the effort.

Sue was a 55 year old female who had put on an extra 50 pounds during the middle age period of her life. She told me she was looking in the mirror one day and just hated how she looked. Her cholesterol was also elevated and she had recently started taking blood pressure medicine. That morning she said she had had enough. She was determined to lose the extra weight and get her blood pressure and cholesterol under control. A plan for her eating was developed as well as an exercise program which consisted of daily walking and toning exercises. The weight came off slowly but today Sue is 60, looks great and not only walks but also runs regularly as part of her exercise program. Her eating and exercise habits are now just part of her life and she says she wouldn't change them for anything.

Patty, another woman in her 50s, had gained weight since going through menopause and taking hormone replacement therapy. She felt the hormones made her hungry and were part of the reason she gained weight. Patty made the decision to stop taking the hormones. After doing this, she was able to get her appetite under control and was able to reduce the amount of food she was consuming everyday. Patty did not go on an exercise program. She and her husband own several acres of land and farm it in the summer. She said she got plenty of exercise working in the garden and taking care of the farm. Patty says she weighs less today than when she graduated from high school. I don't know how much weight she lost but she looks good!

Julie was a 24 year old African American female. She came from a family where most of her family members were obese. She was obese as a child. She says she was miserable as a teenager as she could not participate in many of the activities her friends did and could not wear clothes that were in style as she could not find them in her size. She did not exercise and would often eat second, third and fourth helpings at meals. When she left home to go to college she became good friends with a girl who was going to college on a military schlorship. Her friend was very blunt with her about her weight. Julie began to exercise with her friend and reduce her portion sizes when she ate. As she lost weight and became more physically fit she discovered she enjoyed exercise. In fact, she enjoyed her new lifestyle so much; she changed her major in college to exercise physiology. Not only did she graduate from college, but she graduated with a beautiful figure and with a career that would help keep her physically fit for life.

I've seen many people turn their life around by changing the way they eat and exercise. But I've also seen those who don't. One woman wanted to lose weight so badly.

She would cry when I saw her at the clinic because of her weight. We had many conversations about what she could do to lose weight. She even lived next to a park that had a three mile walking trail on the grounds. For some reason she just could never make the decision to change her lifestyle habits. Don't let this happen to you. Make your plan and live your plan and turn your life around. You can if you think you can.

If it is to be, it is up to me.

Chapter Thirteen

You Can if You Think You Can

Very few of us like or are comfortable with change. We all have our comfort zones, and change takes us out of our comfort zones into the unknown. Change is not always easy. There are challenges associated with change. We are often afraid of change. If we can get past the obstacles we face with change, we can change and hopefully make our lives better. Remember, obstacles are what you see when you take your eyes off your goals.

To make changes in your life, to lose weight and live a healthier lifestyle, you need to take a very objective look at your life and what you are doing and make the decision on what you need to change. It will require effort and work, but it will be worth it. It may be hard to do, but it will be worth it. It will require a clear knowledge of where you want to be, and it will be worth it. It will require discipline, patience, commitment and focus, and it will be worth it.

Make your decision to change and move forward now. Decide on your goals, make your plan and move forward now. Put your plan into action. It will be worth it.

Think of the little train going up the hill saying, "I think I can, I think I can, I think I can." Once you crest the top of the hill, it's down hill from there. Your new life changes will become your norm. You will reach the bottom of the hill with a smile on your face and be able to say, "I knew I could!"

Good luck! I know you can do it! You can if you think you can!

I would love to hear your success stories. Don't hesitate to write or email me at:

Teresa Blanc
6710 Sherman Rd.
Atchison, KS 66002

teresa@teresablancworld.com

When you look in the mirror every morning, you are looking at the person who is responsible for your future.

Remember, if you don't start, you never finish.

Stay focused!!

Never, never quit!!

Appendix

<u>WEIGHT LOSS GRAPH</u>
(Fig. One)

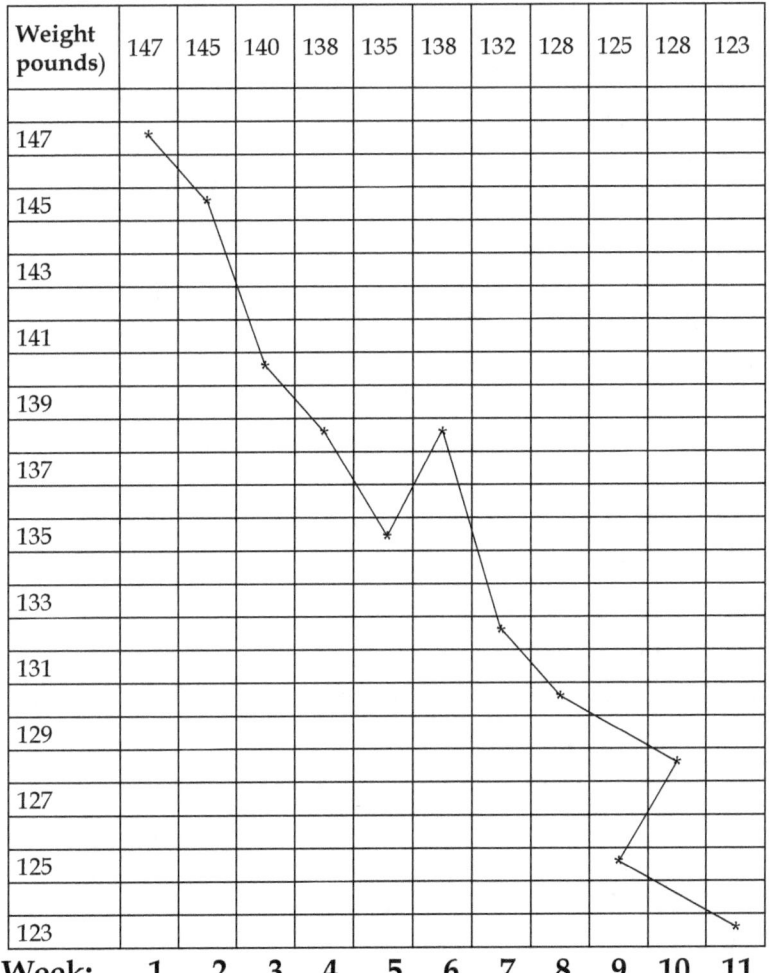

Weight pounds)	147	145	140	138	135	138	132	128	125	128	123

Write your beginning weight in the upper left box. Write in your weekly weights below this and plot them on the graph as each week passes. Connect your dots with straight lines to complete your graph.

WEIGHT LOSS GRAPH
(Fig. 2)

Weight (pounds)										

Week: 1   2   3   4   5   6   7   8   9   10   11

Write your beginning weight in the upper left box. Write in your weekly weights below this and plot them on the graph as each week passes.

FOOD & FLUIDS DIARY
(Fig. 3)

Date	Time	Food/ Fluid	Calories	E.D.	Activity while eating	Feelings

<u>REWARDS & BONUSES</u>
(Fig. 4)

WHEN	THEN
1.	
2.	
3.	
4.	
5.	
6.	
7.	
8.	
9.	
10.	
11.	
12.	

SELF-MONITORING
(Fig. 5)

Date:	Week
Weight:	Pounds lost:
Waist:	Inches lost:
Hips:	Inches lost:
Bust:	Inches lost:
Upper thighs:	Inches lost:
Upper arms:	Inches lost:
Calves:	Inches lost:

DAILY EXERCISE LOG
(Fig. 6)

Date	Type of Activity	Time	Distance/Steps
(example) Monday, 1-1-2008	Walking	30 minutes	535 steps

*One mile = 2,000 to 2,500 steps
10,000 steps = 4 to 5 miles

BODY MASS INDEX (BMI)

WEIGHT POUNDS	HEIGHT								
	4'10"	5'0"	5'2"	5'4"	5'6"	5'8"	5'10"	6'0"	6'2"
125	26	24	23	22	20	19	18	17	16
130	27	25	24	22	21	20	19	18	17
135	28	26	25	23	22	21	19	18	17
140	29	27	26	24	23	21	20	19	18
145	30	28	27	25	23	22	21	20	19
150	31	29	27	26	24	23	22	20	19
155	32	30	28	27	25	24	22	21	20
160	34	31	29	28	26	24	23	22	21
165	35	32	30	28	27	25	24	22	21
170	36	33	31	29	28	26	24	23	22
175	37	34	32	30	28	27	25	24	23
180	38	35	33	31	29	27	26	25	23
185	39	36	34	32	30	28	27	25	24
190	40	37	35	33	31	29	27	26	24
195	41	38	36	34	32	30	28	27	25
200	42	39	37	34	32	30	29	27	26
205	43	40	38	35	33	31	29	28	26
210	44	41	38	36	34	32	30	29	27
215	45	42	39	37	35	33	31	29	28
220	46	43	40	38	36	34	32	30	28
225	47	44	41	39	36	34	32	31	29
230	48	45	42	40	37	35	33	31	30

*BMI is defined as body weight (in kg) divided by height (in m2).

Quick Order Form

Postal orders: Teresa Blanc, 6710 Sherman Rd., Atchison, KS 66002.

Email orders: teresa@teresablancworld.com

Please send the following:

Beat Obesity – You Can if You Think You Can

$13.99 per copy. # copies_____ Total amount:_____

Shipping: Please send $3.00 for the first book and $2.00 for each additional book.

Payment: Cheque or money order.
Credit Card orders: order from web site:
http://teresablancworld.com

Please send more FREE information on:

__Other products ___Speaking/Seminars __Coaching

See http://teresablancworld.com